ACCESS YOUR DRIVE
and ENJOY THE RIDE

ACCESS YOUR DRIVE
and ENJOY THE RIDE

A Guide on Achieving Your Dreams
from a Person with a Disability

LAUREN "LOLO" SPENCER

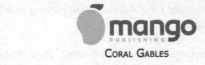

mango
PUBLISHING

CORAL GABLES

Cover Design: Elina Diaz
Cover Photo/illustration: Taj Stansberry
Layout & Design: Elina Diaz

For permission requests, please contact the publisher at:
Mango Publishing Group
2850 S Douglas Road, 2nd Floor
Coral Gables, FL 33134 USA
info@mango.bz

For special orders, quantity sales, course adoptions and corporate sales, please email the publisher at sales@mango.bz. For trade and wholesale sales, please contact Ingram Publisher Services at customer.service@ingramcontent.com or +1.800.509.4887.

Access Your Drive and Enjoy the Ride: A Guide on Achieving Your Dreams from a Person with a Disability

Library of Congress Cataloging-in-Publication number: 2022946623
ISBN: (print) 978-1-68481-011-6 , (ebook) 978-1-68481-012-3
BISAC category code: BIO033000, BIOGRAPHY & AUTOBIOGRAPHY / People with Disabilities

TABLE OF CONTENTS

INTRODUCTION

"Life is what you make it" is probably one of the most common sayings someone throws at you when you're navigating your experiences. As cliché as the statement is, it's still very true. For instance, I currently star in the TV show *The Sex Lives of College Girls*, on HBO Max; I'm the voice of Jazzy on Disney Jr.'s *Firebuds*; I'm an Independent Spirit Award-nominated actress; I've modeled for top brands like Tommy Hilfiger Adaptive and Lady Foot Locker; I have been on panels from Adobe to Cannes Lions; I own a lifestyle brand called Live Solo and run a social media brand; and I do it all from the comfort (and sometimes discomfort) of my wheelchair. With the type of career I've created in the past seven-plus years, not a single soul could've told me anything that I'm doing now was possible for someone with a disability.

Society has never been in support of people with disabilities' dreams. We aren't taught about disability in history books; we are conditioned to ignore people with disabilities from the moment we enter the classroom as six-year-olds. Kids with disabilities rode a different bus, they studied in a whole different section of the school, and they played at different times than everyone else. This pattern of complete avoidance toward people with disabilitiese follows us all through primary and high school into adulthood, when we get to go to college. College is a free-for-all of learning at the higher level, but in my opinion, it's more beneficial in learning who *you* are. And if you're a person with disability who was either born disabled or acquired a disability at a young age—like myself—when you finally become an adult, you are all of a sudden thrown into the world with everyone else. You're now wondering, "How am I supposed to figure this part of life out?", when all your earlier life was spent being ignored or limited. This is the experience of the vast majority of people living with disabilities. So, when people witness the sort of career I've accomplished, everyone is eager to know, "*How* did you accomplish a career like this?" But I was being asked my "how" long before I even thought of a career in front of the camera.

Ever since I started creating a social circle of friends in college, people had always encouraged me to "tell my story," perceiving that my story, for some reason, was so fascinating that it needed to be shared with others. But when people told me that I should share my story, I would always draw a blank— not because I felt like my life was insignificant, but because I just never understood what it was about my story that people wanted to know so badly. Why does everyone seem fascinated with my life? My life isn't much different from yours. Well, I know I am a wheelchair user, but *still!* It's challenging to even consider that it's because of my disability that people have shown interest in knowing the depths of my life, because it's rarely the first thing I think about when sharing who I am. So here is the short version, to get it out the way.

My journey with disability began when I was fourteen years old, diagnosed with ALS (amyotrophic lateral sclerosis, a.k.a. Lou Gehrig's disease)—although that is up for question, since the life expectancy of an ALS patient is five to seven years from diagnosis and yet, twenty years later, I'm very much alive and well. However, as a result of whatever this diagnosis may be, I have lost muscle strength and muscle mass over time. I'm currently in my mid-thirties, and now I'm an ambulatory wheelchair user. An ambulatory wheelchair user is someone who uses a wheelchair as a mobility device, but still has the ability to stand and walk. I wanted to explain that because, like I said earlier, most of us learn the stereotype of disability and wheelchair users—is that you're completely paralyzed if you have to use one— which is not true at all.

My experiences navigating my teenage into adulthood years have been full of many lessons, especially doing it all as a person with a disability. These lessons all boiled down to one underlying action. Applying this action has led me to spend that past seven-plus years developing a successful career in the entertainment industry, and uninhibitedly acting as a disability advocate at the same time. Was this the "plan"? No, but once I recognized that my social media content was making a difference in other people's lives, I knew there was more to my work than just shooting videos and posting. Since then, I have developed a lifestyle brand called Live Solo, dedicated to supporting young adults with disabilities in achieving independence and self-empowerment; started a video production company called Sitting Pretty Productions; and I'm in the early stages of developing a nonprofit organization. This now leads me back to where I left off. Why do people want me to tell my story?

When I think of this question, it always leads me to some deep thinking and self-reflection. When I was first really pushed to answer this, I came up with an answer: "People want to know my story because they can't figure out how someone with a disability who's a wheelchair user can be incredibly happy and fruitful in life!" But, once I got my emotional frustration out of the way I also figured, maybe people want to know because they've never interacted with a person with a disability and are curious, or maybe they've recognized their own non-disabled privilege and want allyship, or maybe people just want to know straight from the source how I achieved my current lifestyle—disability or not. It's challenging to know people's reasons for wanting to know my story because, too many times throughout my life, the question always came with an undertone of assumption that being disabled and being happy are things that cannot coexist. How fucked-up is that? You mean to tell me that you believe that people with disabilities (15 percent of the world's population) can't be happy with their lives? Is it *that* bad? But when I have talked to many people, disabled and non-disabled alike, from all backgrounds, of all ages, genders, etc., I learned that people with disabilities really didn't know how to live with their disability and be happy, or people didn't know that happy people with disabilities existed. This perception of the disability lifestyle was destructively skewed to be so overwhelmingly negative that, when people saw or met me, they assumed I must've cracked life's code in a way that many haven't figured out, whether disabled or not, and so people are eager to know what I did.

This was my thought process behind the content I created on my YouTube channel, *Sitting Pretty*. I would show people all the positive, fun, dope things I did in life to show that disability lifestyle can be fun, fly, and sexy, just like anything else. But was that the reason why people wanted to know my story? My positivity? Something about it felt semi-true, but I felt there was something more meaningful about my story than just my positivity. I reframed the question this time from *Why do people want me to tell my story?* to *What about my story do people want me to tell that they can apply to their lives, too? What is my cheat code to life?* When brainstorming from this perspective, I came up with what is now revealed throughout this book.

For me, life's code goes back to that moment when I realized that my success had boiled down to that one underlying action I mentioned earlier. This action is something we do all day long, but mostly with no self-awareness. But what happens to your life when you take this action and add intention and understanding to it? The action I use that determines *everything* I accomplish: I make decisions.

That's it.

Every extreme turning point, every experience, "good" or "bad," all boiled down to making a decision. A very simple, basic thing, but somehow, it's the toughest thing for people to do. The tough part of making a decision is that you can't guarantee that the decision you make is the right one for you, at any given time in your life, and that's scary. But decision-making isn't about right or wrong. It's more of a this-or-that scenario. Any decision we make is never meant to harm us; in fact, every decision we make is for our betterment, because at the core, decision-making always equates to momentum in your life. If you're not making decisions, you're not moving in life. No matter the direction, you are not creating experiences, lessons, or success by staying still. Everyone's journey is different, and, if you are of any age with at least some self-awareness, you can admit that every memorable experience was the result of a major decision that, whether it was immediately or later, taught you a lesson that propelled your life to continue past those moments.

I'm no saint. I'm no professional scholar. I've made decisions against my better judgment that came with consequences. I made decisions that, on the surface, made absolutely no sense that, surprisingly, came with rewards. But no matter the decision, it never came with a regret. It wasn't always easy, but it became easier over time.

This book is a collection of real stories from my life that made all the difference in the direction my life went, based on making decisions. My hope is that, through my experiences with making pivotal decisions, you'll be empowered to make those decisions in the best way for your own life. To not lead with fear or anxiety because we can't predict the outcomes of our decisions before we make them, but instead to see every decision as an opportunity for an experience to make you grow and move you closer to the desires of your heart. That, although we can't guarantee the result, we can reframe it to understand that, regardless of which decision we make, the unknown is always working to our benefit along with our intentions. So life is what you make it, thanks to your decisions.

Chapter 1

NAH, NOT ME

"Die in five to seven years?! Absolutely not!"

When I was six years old, a few years after my parents divorced, my mom, sister, and I moved to Stockton California from Los Angeles. Stockton was one of those towns where everyone knows everyone, even intergenerationally. My friends' parents were childhood friends with my mom. You could end up making a new friend in school and later find out you're technically blood cousins. Stockton was large enough that you could stay on your side of town and never really venture off to other parts of town your entire life, if you wanted. It's a place full of humble beginnings I appreciate to the fullest. I knew it was where I wanted to be when we took our first visit to K-Mart after moving from LA and ran into one of my six uncles and my cousin. When my cousin and I learned we were going to be at the same elementary school together, we were elated. I liked this place already!

I recognize now that my mother's decision to do what was best for my sister and me, at the sacrifice of what she wanted, changed the trajectory of our well-being forever. My mom was always a person who moved to the beat of her own drum. Those who know her know that my mom does not play when it comes to her kids. I remember one time having a conversation with her about my friend who traveled the world alone, in which she told me, "There is no way I could handle you or your siblings traveling the world solo. My heart couldn't take it. I'd have to go with you guys." That's the kind of mom she is. We have always come first to her, sometimes even before herself. But if you ask her, she wouldn't have it any other way. She was never able to spoil us with material things—we just didn't have it like that. But she spoiled us with her love and support. Not one game, dance performance, or award ceremony was ever missed. My mother decided to put our interests first, and her decision laid the foundation of morals I carried with me through my experiences growing up.

We grew up in our maternal grandparents' home, where playtime with my cousins was a constant lit-ass time. I was very physically active as a kid. We ran around the house like wild, sliding down the stairs on slippery cushions, and running back up the stairs to do it all over again. We didn't get away with this for too long, though, because Grandpa would come around the corner and yell at us to stop before we hurt ourselves. We were constantly in the pool and bunked in the living room when we got to have sleepovers together. Each of us would have our own sleeping bag and wear Grandpa's old t-shirts as pajamas. We put on fashion shows and dance routines for our parents when they came home from work. In the afternoons, when our grandparents babysat us, we ran Fortune 500 companies with our grandma's old briefcases and legal notepads with "meeting notes" scribbled all over them. Imagination was fully encouraged within my family, since our family is rooted in creativity, especially music and performing. My grandpa is revered as one of the best saxophonists who ever lived, one uncle is an award-winning drummer, two uncles perform together on the Las Vegas Strip (one on saxophone, the other on trumpet), and another is a DJ, while my sister was a hip-hop dancer and my younger brother (who was born shortly after we moved to Stockton) played piano and made beats while he was in middle school.

Oh, and everybody sings. Attending live shows growing up was normal for me. Witnessing my family on stage in front of crowds of people, singing, dancing, smiling, and having fun, was something special that I knew the average person didn't have the talent to do. It was their superpower, and it made me proud to be part of the family.

By the time I started high school, I didn't see myself on any stages. I didn't have any superpowers (so I thought at the time). I had accepted myself as the normal one in my family. I was more brown-skinned than my mom and sister. I had shorter, kinkier hair that my mom did her best to manage with Just For Me perm kits and hot rollers every morning, and I had a gap-toothed smile that I loved. All I wanted to do was go to school, hang out with friends, talk about my unhealthy obsession with B2K, and become a journalist. I didn't need to be on stage like the rest of my family. I decided to accept myself as naturally different from my family, which was truly a subconscious decision, because it had nothing to do with any negative influence from my family or friends at all. After observing everyone I was around, I'd found where it made sense for me to exist as the teenager I was. At this time, my mom was renting her first house: a humble house, full of love and good times, that was all her own. Life was good to me, but a very random incident would shake up my world completely.

One night, my mom called us to the kitchen to make our plates for dinner. I rushed into the kitchen, grabbed a dinner plate from a top cabinet with my right hand, and, once I gripped the plate, my entire arm dropped to the counter. I stopped in pure confusion because I felt my arm drop, but the plate was still gripped in my hand. I didn't drop the plate, but it seemed as if the plate weighed five hundred pounds. I knew something was wrong, but I couldn't make any sense of it. I didn't know what to do. I just stood there looking down at my arm in confusion, like, *How did I just do that? Am I trippin'? I know I felt my arm drop, but the plate is in my hand. This is weird. Maybe I'm trippin.'* Then I went to the table as usual. I knew better than to bring up something that might be wrong to my mother unless I was positively sure of how I felt, because she would get concerned. I didn't want to scare her, so I kept it to myself. Although I was scared, I felt there was nothing I could do, so I brushed it off, hoping it was just a one-time occurrence.

According to my mom, when I did finally tell her something different was happening to my body, I was telling her how I'd noticed I couldn't jump as high as I felt I should have been able to when I was in gym class. She knew it was a real concern for me, and in true Mom mode, she took me to see a doctor. However, neither one of us could've predicted that visit would be the start of a more-than-a-year-long journey where we would continue to go from doctor to doctor. My mom later told me that, for her, it felt strange that the doctors never seemed to have an answer regarding my sudden change in physical strength, but she knew she needed to figure out what was happening, even if that meant having to go visit another doctor or do another test. She was determined. My fourteen-year-old brain was not concerned at all about what was going on. This was actually a fun time for me. At fourteen, any reason to go to school late or leave early, spend the day with my mom, and have lunch "off-campus" (a huge luxury as a high school freshman) was a win, even if it was only to go to the doctor. I had no idea of the seriousness of what was really happening. Truthfully, I believe my mom was intentional in making the experience feel like a regular day and a regular visit to prevent me from being scared over something we didn't have an answer for. She knew how important it was to make sure this was a positive experience for me, because her priority as a mother was to always make the best decision for the well-being of her kids.

The decisions we make as individuals will always impact those around us, whether we intend them to or not—it's inevitable. As Einstein said, "Energy cannot be created or destroyed; it can only be changed from one form to another." This applies to human behavior as well. My mom's decision to keep this slew of inconclusive doctor visits as normal as possible impacted my experience and shielded me from having a negative or fearful reaction to what was happening, so that I can now, as an adult, look back at that time and remember it as something fun.

As an adult, looking back, I honor my mom's bravery during this time because I know this process affected her deeply, but she never showed it. She stayed diligent in seeking some sort of answer for the inexplicable changes happening in my body. Test after test, this MRI, that blood test, this "exercise," that EMG test (these were the worst), time and time again. My mom witnessing my limbs grow weaker instead of stronger was mind-boggling, followed by no real answers and accompanied by no explanations. Then we started making visits to the University of California, San Francisco (UCSF) on a regular basis. This was the first time we visited the same place more than once, and I knew there must be something they knew that other doctors didn't. The drive was long, and the visit even longer. We would be there almost six hours seeing every type of doctor you could imagine, each of them doing their own special tests on me. Still clueless about what was really happening, I was just trying to stay entertained during the visit, since social media did not exist back then.

After some time spent going on a rat race for an answer from what felt like every type of doctor Northern California had to offer, my mom called me into her room from watching

TV. Immediately, my mind raced to recall anything that could've happened earlier that day that I could be getting in trouble for, since that was the usual reason she would call one of us to her room. Whatever it was, I was going to have my reason why I didn't deserve to be in trouble. When I walked in, she was sitting up in her bed with her bathrobe, pajamas, and glasses on. Her Bible was open, and she had a highlighter in hand with a concordance sitting beside her. This was her nighttime routine. She closed her Bible, moved the concordance, and told me to sit next to her in bed. And she said:

"You know how we've been going doctor to doctor all this time, and to San Francisco?"

"Yeah."

"Well, the doctors believe they have an answer to what's been going on."

I stayed silent.

"They say you have ALS."

I stayed silent.

"Do you know what that is?"

I shook my head.

She proceeded to explain what "ALS" stood for, and that it was a condition where my muscles would weaken as I grew older. She offered a rather simplified explanation, one my fourteen-year-old self could understand.

I stayed silent throughout her explanation.

"What are you thinking?"

I shrugged. "Can I go watch TV now?"

She smiled. "Yes, you can."

That was it. I had no reaction, because I was fourteen. I kind of didn't care. It was like, "Cool, now we know, but hurry up, Mom. I'm trying to get back to watching TV with my brother." The weight and severity of what my mom was telling me about my body somehow didn't translate in that moment. It didn't hit me that my new "diagnosis" was something serious until my grandparents, stepdad, sister, and biological dad came into town, and we all went on a road trip to UCSF together. What were once just regular road trips with my mom turned into a caravan excursion with my whole immediate family. When we arrived at the facility, I was escorted into one of the patient rooms as usual, while everyone else, including my mom, went to the head doctor's office. I knew it was something serious, and that it was about me, because I was never left in a patient room alone. About an hour later, my sister came into the room to get me and take me to where the rest of the family was waiting, which was no longer in the doctor's office. They were all on a completely different floor of the facility. When we got there, the only people left were my grandparents. I saw my stepdad and biological dad at the other end of the floor, separate from everyone, and I had no idea where my mom had gone. My sister proceeded to tell me what had happened.

What happened in the doctor's office is something I will not be sharing with you all because of its personal nature, and because I want to keep this sacred to my family, but let's just say, to a room full of adults who love you dearly, hearing news like an ALS diagnosis is bound to cause kneejerk reactions. The car ride home was much less lively than it had been on the way there. Next, a huge "family meeting" happened at the house. All of my uncles and aunts came over and piled into the living room. When my family calls a "family meeting," we know it is something serious, because it is strictly for the adults while the kids stay outside. This time, however, my cousins didn't come over. It was just me waiting separately, by myself, just as I had done when we went to UCSF. That's how I knew it was about me and whatever the doctors had told my family at the facility.

I learned more recently that the doctors recommended my immediate family meet with them before the whole family could know. The mood the doctors tried to create with my family was what they knew based on their experiences with other patients. My diagnosis was accompanied with a life expectancy of five to seven years, and doctors said my family needed to prepare for the worst and what life could look like moving forward for them and me. My mom couldn't explain that to my extended family on her own. She needed support to figure out what to do and how to handle this news, so much so that, once she knew, it was weeks before she even told me of my diagnosis. She said she had needed time to process what the doctors had told her. The initial news broke her down completely, but she could never show it because she knew it would affect me. Instead, she made the decision to watch me. She noticed how much fun I was having as a young girl. How I was always laughing at something and goofing around with my brother and sister and all the friends I was constantly around. She knew she couldn't accept the news from the doctor. She respected their expertise, but her gut told her I wasn't going to die young. She made the decision that this diagnosis was not going to change how she would love or treat me, or how anyone else in the family would love or treat me. She was going to do it her way—the way God told her to handle it.

Once my entire family was made aware of my diagnosis, my mom and I continued our visits to UCSF. As before, we went every six months for my checkups for the next three years straight, faithfully. Doctor after doctor, test after test, all day tracking my progress. Every doctor would always say, "You're holding up well. You're in great shape. *Wow!*" This was always great because it meant nothing had really changed, which left them baffled after seeing me. Not being sure what type of results they were expecting, I didn't care how they felt. Hearing them congratulate me on my progress during every visit caused me to become curious as to why me being in good health was such a monumental moment for the doctors. Until that moment, all I knew was that my muscles would get weaker over time. Big deal. I had my whole life to live before something like that happened. The way those doctors looked confused after seeing me was a sign that there was more to this diagnosis that I wasn't understanding.

At home by myself, I was on the computer waiting for the dial-up internet to boot my AOL, in the old-school and very slow way the internet worked back in the day. When I finally connected to the internet, I searched on ALS. I was ready to learn what I felt everyone else knew about my diagnosis except me. A bunch of links came up, and I just clicked the one that looked the most credible, one ending in ".org." I skimmed through until I saw the list of symptoms of ALS. The muscle weakness in my limbs was what I had been experiencing, so no surprise there. Then the symptoms got more severe. I read that I could lose strength in my tongue such that I would struggle to speak, or lose strength in my eyelids such that I wouldn't be able to open my eyes on my own, and that most people were dead within five to seven years of diagnosis. I stopped reading. I closed the browser and shut the computer down. It was in this moment that I made the first decision for myself, the same way my parents had to do when I was younger. It was the biggest decision of my life because of the way it affected my mind, body, and experiences forever. This decision was so powerful I had no idea how far it would take me or how impactful it would be until years later.

I made the decision that what I had just read online about ALS was *not* going to be my life. I would never accept the effects of this diagnosis as my truth. My mind immediately shifted to everything that was the opposite of what the internet tried to say was going to happen to me. *Die in five to seven years?! Absolutely not!* Nah, not me. I didn't have any specific plan. I just became determined to prove the internet wrong, to prove doctors wrong, and to prove to myself that I had much more life to live, and I became determined to live it to the fullest. Everything in my spirit told me what I had read was a lie regarding my life. My future was filled with too many things I still had to achieve. My imagination was too big for what that article tried to tell me was going to happen to me. I was not going out like that. I still had to go to college, get my first boyfriend, become a famous journalist, travel the world, run my company, like I did when I played pretend as a kid.

My mind raced. Everything in my chest and spirit suddenly felt like it stood ten times higher, all with this strong sense of certainty that I was right in my decision. No doctor, no adult, no internet, no person could tell me otherwise. I never looked up what ALS meant again. I knew all I needed to know, and now I was choosing to focus on creating the life I'd always dreamed of and making it a reality.

Society has always made living with a disability a death sentence for your dreams and desires. People have been conditioned to believe that, once you acquire a disability or are born with one, your possibilities for living the life you desire are over. They shut down the dreams of people with disabilities because of what a doctor might say. There is rarely anyone who approaches disability wanting to find solutions or other opportunities to achieve the same goals while having a disability. Even in that moment, "disability" wasn't what I was escaping—I was deciding to escape death.

Roll It Back

Sometimes we don't realize how much our parents' influence ends up affecting our lives until we reach the age our parents were when they were raising us. How they grew up affected the decisions they made in their lives—that's human nature. But we always have the power to make different decisions than the generations before us. These experiences, whether perceived as good or bad, have the power to shape our decision-making, even at the subconscious level. There are many new decisions being made by millennials in society who are challenging and changing their decisions to better serve their needs. For example, look at the upward trend in entrepreneurship. This generation is learning that you can still achieve a lavish lifestyle and wealth without needing to do the "traditional" go-to-college, get-a-degree, and find-a-job routine passed down from previous generations. People now are even redefining what marriage is to them, or delaying marriage altogether. The "traditional" way was to meet someone nice, be monogamous only, have kids, have the wife stay home while the husband works, and grow old together. Now, people are practicing different marriage styles like polyamory, women are proud to build careers and juggle motherhood, men are open to being house husbands, and people are more willing to wait to marry until they are truly ready. Prioritizing mental health has been one of the most prominent new decisions made by millennials. If you've ever been to a therapy session, you know that one of the first things a therapist wants to dissect is your childhood. Those are our roots, and those roots are the foundation for how strong and independent we grow. Breaking generational curses is the result of adults making the decision to create "new roots" for their futures based on their dissatisfaction with the way they grew up. Because it's a fact that, if they don't decide to break the "curse," decisions from previous generations will continue to be passed down until someone does make the decision to change it.

Keeping a positive perspective creates the opportunity to make decisions with your own best interest at heart first. Whether you inherited positivity from others, like I did from my mom, or it's a skillset you must learn from scratch—either way, it is the key to living the life you desire. It's not a skill you master overnight, and even if you witness another person using it, you must still learn to master it in your own way, within your own timing. While I inherited positive thinking from my mom's conscious and subconscious decision-making, it was the decisions I had to make on my own beyond this point that would determine the direction of my life.

Get Rolling

Setting Up a Positive Foundation for Your Independence

Looking back now, as an adult, I recognize that the only reason I could believe I had the ability to make such a firm, against-the-grain decision was my mother's decision-making. Her energy in approaching my diagnosis in a positive way kept me in a positive space. Her decisions affected me more than I ever knew at that time. It was because of her that I dared to live life to the beat of my own drum, too.

My mom decided that providing a healthier environment, surrounded by love and support from her family, was better for us growing up. This came at the expense of her leaving the city she loved to live in, and being a single mother of two little girls. Meanwhile, my dad, who had his personal struggles, decided to go after his dreams no matter what. This came at the expense of him not being able to easily spend time with his kids. To this day, my parents both agree that, although that time in life was tough, they know they made the right decisions as individuals and as parents. Their inherent sense to make pivotal decisions rooted in what they knew was best has shown its influence upon my own behavior in how I've made my decisions. Their influence, which was completely unintentional, led me to recognize that, no matter the circumstances I'm in, I must always choose what is best for me regardless of any fear, outside perception, or new circumstance I didn't expect to experience. As long as I know I'm doing my best, that's all the confirmation I need to carry me into the next phase in life's journey.

Practicing Positivity

Before making a decision, switch up your point of view. Here are some ways I approach positivity when making a decision:

1. **Choose joy.** Even if you feel fear, luckily, you have the chance to choose the opposite, which is joy. Remember, energy can only be changed from one form to another, so make the decision to change from fear to joy. Being in a joyful energy space breeds positive experiences.

2. **Patience is key!** Take time to think about your decision and process the problem. Find the positive solution and move forward in that direction.

3. **Trust yourself over society.** Society doesn't have all the answers. Be real with yourself, listen to your gut, and release judgment!

4. **Be intentional in all your decisions.** Have a clear understanding as to why you are making a decision, and use that intention as your moral compass moving forward.

Setting Up Your Foundation

Take a second to think about your foundation. Not all families are perfect, but think about the people you love and admire in your life—whether it's a parent, grandparent, sibling, or friend. Do you admire their positivity, gratitude, or compassion?

Here are questions to ask yourself with regard to your foundation:

1. Who do I consider a part of my foundation? What are the traits I most admire about them? How can I implement those behaviors in my life?

2. What are generational curses around me? What can I do to overcome them?

3. Who from my foundation can I ask for support in moving forward with this decision?

Chapter 2

WHAT'S ACCESSIBILITY?

"My wheelchair gave me freedom."

Many people would consider something like this happening to me at such a young and pivotal age to be unfortunate. Because I've made it all the way through adulthood and am still thriving, I'm glad the initiation of this experience happened at age fourteen. When you're a teenager, you get to take advantage of the "ignorance is bliss" way of thinking. Many things roll off your shoulders because your young mind can't quite comprehend severe experiences. Yet, you're still old enough to make decisions for yourself, and adults must consider your perspective.

Going back to school, now as a student with a disability, shifted how I experienced classes the remainder of my high school years. Between myself, my mom, and my high school counselor, we were able to put together a plan to make my time as a student as seamless as possible while maintaining a positive social experience. I made it very clear to my counselor that I did not want to start taking the small yellow bus to school. I didn't want to be separated from my friends because the school gave me the option to start going to the—I hate this term—"special needs" class. I wanted to simply continue going to school like I always had, but with some minor adjustments here and there when needed. It was important for me to make that decision for myself, because I was focused on the life I wanted to live, not the one society created for me without my consent. That's where the mark is missed constantly when handling accessibility accommodations for teens and young adults with disabilities.

Lawmakers and people of power never consider the lives of those with disabilities that they are affecting and have convinced themselves they're helping. They immediately go with their marginalizing way of thinking. This means they are influenced by negative attitudes associated with the disabled experience, and they make decisions based on those assumptions. They never consider or attempt to reach out to the disabled community on what we need and how we want things to happen for us. Luckily, I had my counselor and my mom, who made sure to consult with me on what I needed and made sure it happened that way, instead of saying "Now that you're disabled, you have to do things this way only." It was just as important to them that I live the life I desired as it was for me to have the experiences I wanted. Your foundation of supporters is crucial to your well-being in anything that you do. When I finally had the courage to ask my mom what her response was to the doctors after they told her about my diagnosis, she said:

"I broke down. Hearing the news of your child only having two to five years to live was devastating. But it was something I could never accept. It was like I heard what they said, but I knew I wasn't supposed to throw in the towel. I watched you for a couple of weeks before I even told you about your diagnosis. I saw how loved you were by your friends, how happy you always were, and you always had a big spirit with a positive aura. I told myself, 'If she's good then I'm good.' I knew, after seeing that, that whatever the doctors thought could happen to you was not going to be your story. God had a plan for you, and all my job was to make sure I supported you as much as I had the power to, and make sure you lived. I wasn't going to change anything about our lifestyle as a family or the way we treated you because of the doctor's news. It was because of your energy, daughter, that everyone else who was around you naturally fell in line."

You must begin to pay attention and become selective about who you allow yourself to be around and who you allow to influence your life decisions. Had my mom, or any of my family and friends, followed what the doctors said instead of how they genuinely felt, who knows how my life would've turned out. The energy from their positive thoughts directly affected my responses to my changing health without my even knowing it. I knew that I had to start making decisions about who I was going to be around because I had the awareness, even as a teen, to know that the people who loved me unconditionally were who I needed to keep living my life. Anyone who wasn't aligned with that, I never could stay close with for too long.

There were multiple accommodations made on my behalf, thanks to the support of my counselor. One of the best was not having to work out during gym class. I still had to attend, but I would just sit on the side and cheer everyone else on as they were doing their workouts. My teachers started to allow me a grace period to get to my classes, I no longer had to carry my books, and my guidance counselor appointed a designated friend to escort me to my classes because I was still walking around campus (using a wheelchair wasn't necessary yet). I also had a left-handed desk in all of my classes because lefties are the best, a friend took notes for me in every class, and between my friends who had cars, the school nurse, and a teacher whose daughter I grew up with, all would coordinate who could take me home after school. I always felt even cooler when my older sister or one of her friends would pick me up after school, because they would be blasting music super loud out of the car, and they were all beautiful to look at. Rides home with the school nurse were fun too, because she would let me listen to whatever CD I wanted, and she sometimes would take the long way home when there was a song I wanted to hear on repeat that I knew my mom would not allow me to listen to in the house. Rides with my friends were always the best (and scariest) because we had a sense of freedom and maturity. They were also all-new drivers, so close-call accidents happened more than enough times, but luckily, we always made it home safe.

My community of people at school really banded together during this time. I'm not sure if any of my friends officially knew what was going on, but truthfully it didn't matter to them. All these accommodations I looked at as being dope. I liked the changes. Even when I got my AFOs (ankle-foot orthoses)—I called them my Forrest Gump leg braces at the time, since I didn't know the technical name for them—I was excited about them. I thought they were dope because no one else on campus had them. When my friends asked me about them, I would just tell them, "They help me walk better and not trip over my feet." They'd respond, "Cool," and we'd go on about our conversation.

The beautiful thing about this time was that I was well aware of the physical changes and, although the help I was getting from my family, friends, school nurse, and guidance counselor grew exponentially, attitude-wise, nothing changed. My friends were now holding my books on the way to class while we had heated debates about who was the finest member of B2K. I didn't have to make my own plate anymore, but I still couldn't leave the table until I ate all my food. It felt like everyone somehow knew what their part was in helping me, but none of the plan was ever discussed out loud. Not that anyone was hiding it, but no one talked about it either (and, in fairness, I never asked). That was my self-assigned responsibility during this process. I was to simply stay happy because everyone was doing so much for me without needing any level of compensation. I fell into a superhuman complex, which I've learned through my advocacy work is actually called internalized ableism. Internalized ableism is essentially when a person with a disability feels they need to present as "non-disabled" as possible to either fit in to whatever social environment they're surrounded by, or to avoid the reality that they are actually disabled. In my case, I would feel guilty if I expressed any emotional "weakness" or complaint. This can be very detrimental thinking if you're not careful, because it rides a fine line between being courageous and lacking self-love. This was my own doing, nothing pressured by anyone in my foundation. I just never wanted to add anything else to what those in my foundation were already doing so graciously. I couldn't add tears, bad feelings, insecurities, and fear to their plate on top of the rest. I felt I had to fight those feelings by finding positivity and joy in everything in order to protect them.

Putting everyone else's feelings first, before my own, because of my internalized ableism became a common unhealthy theme that would follow me well into adulthood. At the core, internalized ableism isn't a healthy mental space for people with disabilities to operate from; however, for me, it did force me to keep myself in as positive a space as I could possibly be. And because my foundation was also made up of positive, happy people, it at least made being happy and staying happy regularly an achievable thing. Making the decision to be happy and grateful kept me in the attitudinal space I needed to be in, especially during the crucial years of teenage life and puberty.

Going to football games on Friday nights, major school rallies around annual events, and dances were all my absolute favorites. I wasn't allowed to go to house parties in high school because Stockton is still a dangerous city, and back then, shootings or fights at parties were far too common. Given my new disability, I had to be sure I only went places where I felt the safest, which was at home or at my high school. My counselor or an appointed staff member was always there to be sure that I was being taken care of during the events I wanted to attend. This level of assured safety allowed me the freedom to live my high school experience to its fullest capacity. Maintaining my social life (teenager style) was imperative to my growth as a person. I was able to learn the social skills needed to interact with people who were non-disabled as well as normalize myself to these environments, creating a standard for what I needed in order to enjoy a public space like a party and still feel safe. All of this would come in handy during my early twenties and beyond.

Once senior year came around, the reality that my safe space of high school would be coming to an end, and the imperative foundation of family, friends, and staff would all be moving in their own directions, was nerve-racking. This transition is tough on lots of teens, but for me, this turned into a "ride it 'til the wheels fall off" moment. I began to prepare for leaving home to attend college, as all of the senior class was encouraged to do. I applied to a couple of universities, but I was more fixated on making the last year of high school my most fun and best year possible. And I did! I went to every formal dance, every football game, and every rally, went to prom, and most importantly, went to the greatest senior-year night of all, Grad Night Disneyland. In California, there is one dedicated night for high school seniors from all over the state to take over Disneyland after hours and enjoy the park and designated events until the early morning hours the next day. This event became an all-hands-on-deck situation. My high school's staff knew I wanted to go, but they had never had to organize accommodations for a disabled student before, and they already knew that me not attending was *not* an option.

The largest hurdle was figuring out how I would navigate a park of that size independently and safely. This led to the school nurse asking if I would be open to using an electric wheelchair just for Grad Night. I had never considered a wheelchair because I'd never needed one before—my AFO braces were working just fine around campus. I wasn't against it, but I was nervous about using it, until they had me test it out at school, and that changed everything. I was overwhelmingly excited! The freedom the wheelchair gave me was remarkable. It relieved the tension my body would feel after wearing my AFOs all day, I could move around much faster, and it felt like a video game, all at the same time. I immediately agreed to using it for Grad Night. On the day of, all the seniors piled onto the charter buses to drive from Stockton to Anaheim—this is a six-to-eight-hour bus ride. I wanted to be on the bus with my friends, so the school nurse followed behind in a separate van that carried the wheelchair because the charter bus was not set up to have me and the wheelchair on it together. Once we arrived at Disneyland, the nurse brought the wheelchair around the bus for me to sit in it. I was a bit nervous, because this was the first time my friends would see me using one, and I didn't know what they would think. The AFOs were one thing, but a wheelchair? That's a whole other thing to accept.

Thinking back, I hate that those feelings were something I even considered. Even with all the support I was already getting, I still felt nervous about people's opinions regarding a wheelchair. Even knowing how much I loved it, others' opinions affected how I would feel about myself. Where did I learn that? Who told us that wheelchairs were these daunting, scary devices that repelled people? Not because those people even have to use it, but because we are conditioned to believe that this is how people are supposed to react. I believe this level of conditioning comes from the imagery we've all subconsciously seen over and over throughout life. Whenever we see wheelchairs, it's usually because someone is injured. Injuries hurt—injuries mean something bad happened to your body, which then means wheelchair = bad. When a pastor is giving a sermon at church and it's a lesson on miracles and they use the wheelchair as a visual for something wrong in your life, you equate wheelchair with bad. And because we don't have enough imagery showcasing wheelchairs in a more desirable way to balance out the negative perceptions, we will forever think of wheelchairs as something no one ever wants to have to use or experience. Then add that I was a teenager at the time who was already struggling with self-image issues—and I'm now being presented with a wheelchair?! Yeah, a chaos of emotions, but when I felt the full, effortless independence of using the electric wheelchair, I knew I never wanted that feeling to go away.

So, despite what my emotions and insecurities were screaming at me regarding the wheelchair, my newfound independence mattered more. That's why my friends are the absolute greatest. When I turned that wheelchair on and started speeding in one direction, my friends cheered me on like I'd won first place in a competition. They were ecstatic for me, not only because it gave me the freedom I needed, but because this meant I could be right alongside them safely throughout the whole night. When we finally went through the check-in process to get into the park, I turned up in that chair. My friends were hopping on the back to ride with me,

I was speeding back and forth and all around the park, and I did donuts in my chair like a streetcar racer would do to show off his wheels. I was the most popular person that night. Kids from the other schools looked on in amazement, and I made some new friends who I still know to this very day. I was so popular from that night that I made my Myspace username "I Do Donuts in My Chair...What y'all know 'bout it." The night was epic, and all because I made the decision to do what was best for my body and not my ego. As a person with a disability, transitioning from ambulating to using a mobility device can be an intimidating experience, mainly because it solidifies that your body is changing in a way that is out of your control, and the social perception of wheelchairs and other mobility devices is never a positive one. I believe that, since my focus was on what the wheelchair meant for my ability to attend the event and have independence and a good time, that took precedence over any ego concerns I might've drummed up if a wheelchair had been introduced to me under other circumstances. The support and excitement from the staff and my friends also confirmed that I'd made the right decision for me. There was nothing I had to feel ashamed about. This device was practical for what it was intended to do, and I loved what it did for me that night and what a wheelchair would do for me in the future. My wheelchair gave me freedom.

Grad Night left me on a high for the remaining weeks of senior year. My school allowed for one final accommodation, which was to have my sister escort me arm-in-arm on graduation day. It was truly a bittersweet moment for me. I knew I was "leaving the nest," that my school staff had done incredibly well at providing for me to make high school the experience I wanted it to be. Their support, their foundation, had set the bar for how I would continue to vet resources I had to use in the future. My friends were the ultimate emotional support, setting the caliber for what friendship truly means. I would use the way they loved, cared, and encouraged me as my barometer for anyone new I would meet in the future to call a friend. The experience of these people showing up for me 100 percent, every day, for the four years I attended high school was what I needed to prepare for the next pivotal decision of my life.

Roll It Back

When we discuss accessibility and freedom as people with disabilities, it's usually met with negativity because it is assumed that any accommodations needed for a person with a disability would be extreme and hard to implement, which is not true. Accessible accommodations already exist, but since they aren't applied everywhere, true accessibility is lacking, and that's the issue. The true way to accomplish accessibility for people with disabilities is through community effort. It's not extreme; we just need the support and willingness of others who want people with disabilities to experience a life of freedom. That was the determining factor during my high school years—the community of people willing to help and provide solutions, coupled with wanting me to live a full high school life. It was just as much my desire as it was for the entire community of people who supported me as well. It's important as a society to prioritize and be serious about supporting the accessibility needs of the disabled community because we *all* will experience disability within our lifetimes. Whether temporarily, permanently, or through growing old, we all experience disability, and since this will be a rare experience to avoid, it's best that society gets to a point where accessibility for all is first priority in order to have full inclusion. As a society, we should band together to make full accessibility a priority. This has been called "universal design," meaning that everything can be made accessible to the disabled. That means that, if everything is accessible for people with disabilities, it's accessible to all, regardless of what level of ability a person may have. We all have the right to access the world, social settings, and wherever else at an equal rate as anyone else. One of the reasons people feel disability is a life of limitations is because society doesn't get on board to help make the world accessible everywhere to everyone. If accessibility was easily and readily available wherever you went, or incorporated in every experience, life wouldn't be limited. Therefore, people would be able to grasp disability lifestyle in a positive way when it's their time to experience it themselves or through a loved one.

Get Rolling

Vetting Your Foundation

Building a foundation of people in your life is just as important as building a foundation in anything else—a business, a house, a social media following, etc. You must build a solid base for anything you desire to be strong and long-lasting.

When creating a foundation of people in your life, I suggest:

1. **Engaging and building with people who match what you feel are your core values in yourself and in others.** For example, if *supporting others* is a value you truly believe you hold and exude to others, then look for the same level, if not greater, *support of others* in those that are around you. If there are people in your life who

have always gone above and beyond to support you, even more than you ever asked for, especially when you needed them the most, those people stay. If there are people who have rarely supported you in tough experiences, or only support when things are going well for you, then keep those at a distance or end the relationships altogether.

2. **It's okay to keep a safe distance from people who have shown up time and time again to hurt us, even if bloodline is shared.** Keeping negative people around can harm both you and the trajectory of your future. We are humans, not superheroes who can keep everyone else's needs ahead of our own. Your foundation will never put you in a position to feel this way.

3. **Your foundation should always want what's best for you.** I learned from a fellow creator who was a painter that, "Once a customer buys your art for a certain price, never lower your prices afterwards. If one person was willing to pay the price, then multiple people will be willing to pay as well." You can apply this idea to selecting the people you want in your foundation. Once one person shows you that they are capable of support, encouragement, positivity, love, etc., then any person who does not bring those qualities does not need to be around. Because, if one person has those qualities, there are multiple people who do as well, and those are who you focus on to build relationships with.

4. **Your foundation should show you examples of how to stay focused on the important things in life.** They

should encourage you daily so that, when you have your vulnerable moments, you have the advice you need and people to lean on when you are being a human being. It's okay to need help from others.

Vetting Your Ego

When I had to make the decision as to whether I should begin using an electric wheelchair, I had to battle my ego. Had I let the conditioned world of negative perceptions of disability get in my way, I would never have experienced a life of freedom. That moment was a real check to my ego, and if we are not careful, our egos can talk us out of some incredible life-changing experiences. Therefore, we must always check our egos before making a decision to be sure they're not getting in the way of our successes.

Here are some questions to ask yourself to check whether your ego is helping you or harming you:

1. **Who am I making this decision for: myself or others?** If it's yourself, then more than likely your ego is there to help you. If it's for others, there's a good chance ego is harming you and you must be careful in your next steps.

2. **Is this decision in line with my core values?** If the answer is yes, then your ego is on your side giving the confidence you need for next steps. If the answer is no, then your ego is setting you up to fail and be hurt in the process.

3. **Will this decision aid me in becoming the best version of myself?** If the answer is yes, then your ego is supporting you by revealing a new way to approach

your desires. If the answer is no, then your ego is lying to you to further strengthen your insecurities.

your desires. If the answer is no, then surrender is your to
you to further search in your inner drive.

Chapter 3

F*CK IT

*"Mom, if what the doctors say about what
will happen to me is true, then let me leave
while I can still take care of a majority of my
needs independently."*

High school was over, and it was time for me to step into true
adulthood for the first time. Being disabled and an adult added
a new level of responsibility that I was ready to take on, on
my own. I didn't desire to live at home forever, but I was in no
rush to leave either. The foundation that was created for me
kept me safe, kept me comfortable. But it was this same sense
of complacency that kept me stagnant. I could tell I wasn't
growing at the rate I felt I wanted to be at that age, and I didn't
know how to fix it. I was stuck in my comfort zone.

Comfort zones are very tricky. At their core, comfort zones
are technically a good thing. By definition, a comfort zone is *a
place or situation where one feels safe or at ease and without
stress*—and for most people, feeling safe and without stress
is what we want every day. However, living in a comfort zone
also creates a life that is on a constant plateau. No forward
movement, no growth, just stuck in the same run-of-the-mill
experience day by day. My first year out of high school, I
attended our local community college. I wasn't accepted to
any of the universities I applied to, and truthfully, my family
wouldn't have been able to afford for me to go without any
scholarship support anyway. I didn't mind it because I was

still able to live at home, which meant all my needs regarding disability were still being met, and many of my friends from my high school plus friends from the other high schools around the city were all attending this community college too. At the time, I felt it was the perfect way to transition from being a high schooler into being an adult, but reflecting back, I recognize that staying was actually the exact thing that kept me stagnant and in a comfort zone.

A comfort zone isn't created to help push you to a new level, it is rooted in the need to feel safe. Often comfort zones aren't created intentionally. It just hits us one day when we realize nothing in our lives has changed. Time has gone by, and the goals we set for ourselves still haven't been accomplished. We reflect and realize our fears have gotten the best of us because taking a chance felt unsafe. But growing into your dreams is not a safe-feeling process. I don't mean safe in the context of experiencing life-threatening danger. I mean it more in the context of fear vs. courage. To make the dreams in your head a reality is an act of courage because you can't predict what will or will not happen on the journey, and that unknowing can feel very unsafe. But at least you still have a chance to accomplish your dream, because you're in motion toward a goal. Whereas if you let fear take over, it will keep you safe, theoretically, because it feels like a more guaranteed way of predicting what will or will not happen to you. But it's like the saying goes: "We fear going after our dreams because of everything we think might go wrong, but what if everything goes right? Wouldn't you want to know what that's like instead?"

My sense of comfort and safety during this time made me not want to achieve much while at community college. I was still hanging with friends recklessly, missing classes, and experiencing the relative freedom of a college atmosphere.

There wasn't much challenging me to reach a new potential, and I knew it and I took advantage of that. My grades were lower than they had ever been, and I knew I wasn't doing my best, nor was I even trying to. I was only going because my friends were there, and my mom couldn't force me to go to class once I got to campus. I mean that respectfully, because trust me, if my mom had laid down the hammer on anything, I was going to be falling right in line. After a year of slacking off, I realized that, deep down, I knew staying in Stockton was not my future. It's not where I dreamed to be after that AOL search at age fourteen. I didn't know exactly where I was supposed to be, but I knew it wasn't at that college or staying in my hometown. Wherever I felt I needed to be, it was somewhere bigger, livelier. I knew I wanted more than what Stockton could offer me. When a moment like this arises, it's a sign that you need to break out of a comfort zone. You have to begin planning and researching what you could do next. Once you tap into this feeling, it is something you can't ignore—you must follow through. Otherwise, that gut feeling of the need to push through your comfort will haunt you until you make the first step toward the dream. And that first step always begins with a making a decision. My decision was to move to Los Angeles—alone.

My early Los Angeles roots started to rise in my spirit. It was a place that I felt comfortable enough to live in, although I hadn't been back since we moved when I was a little girl. After a long time away, somehow the city still felt familiar. It was still close enough to Stockton for my mom, family, and friends to easily visit me, and I had a plethora of opportunities to create that dream life I had on repeat inside of my head. It was the perfect next step.

I played around with this idea for months, and once I got my final semester transcripts with the lowest GPA I'd ever had, I knew it was time to take the next step and move to Los Angeles. The vision I had for myself at this time was to be a successful journalist. I had written for my high school newspaper and was a journalism major. I've always been obsessed with knowing people's stories and crafting them in a way that was entertaining, yet educational. I wanted to live on my own to prove to myself that I could do it, but was realistic enough to know I needed some type of caregiver to start. But that was too much to think of at the time. LA was my best option for the possibility of my dreams as a journalist being realized, and since it's one of the largest cities in the world for creatives and those who want to be part of the entertainment or media industries, it was a challenging enough place for me to move to and grow in.

Without a real plan in sight, just my gut feeling and the talking points I felt I needed to convince my mom to let me move, I went straight to her. Here's the thing about my mom: you can't give her an idea without a plan, because she knows that whatever her kids are drumming up in their heads, she's going to have to be the most responsible one and put out the money to make it happen. You can't come to her with some bullshit that doesn't add up to her. My talking points were: 1) LA is close, 2) top universities with journalism programs were there, like UCLA, USC, and Cal State Northridge, and 3) the LA Times, and essentially every other major news station or publication, had offices out there, which meant long-term employment after graduating. These were basic points, yet effective, in my mind. Either way, I knew it was now or never. I walked out of my room and into the kitchen, where Mom was going through mail. This conversation was crucial for me if I wanted to make my move happen. I made my next big decision. I walked up to her and said:

"Mom, I need to move out. I need to leave Stockton."

"What do you mean? Where is this coming from?"

"Mom, I'm not being challenged staying here. My grades are terrible. My dreams don't fit here. I need to go to LA."

A surprised look covered my mom's face. It was time to pitch my plan.

"I can go to LA, finish community college out there, transfer to a four-year university there, get a job, then see what happens after that."

As if life was ever that simple, especially for a person with a disability. When you want to live life independently with a disability, you must think of, not only traditional living responsibilities, but also all it takes to maintain our health. Depending on your disability, you could have to think about expenses for medication, accessible housing and mobility equipment, accessibility in neighborhoods, transportation options if you don't drive, live-in vs. visiting caregivers for hygiene support, employment that *must* include full benefits, and much more. Unfortunately, we don't have the option to just pick any place to stay and work multiple random jobs to hustle our way to our dreams like the average person.

"Why don't you just work to get your grades up out here, finish one more year, then transfer to a four-year out there?"

"But they have community colleges in LA. I can just go to one of those. Stockton just isn't for me anymore, Mom."

Not responding, a look of slight fear and hesitation, overcame her. And then I shared the truth behind the urgency.

"Mom, if what the doctors say about what will happen to me is true, then let me leave while I can still take care of a majority of my needs independently, Let me go to LA, live my life to the fullest capacity, and if at any point I need your help to take care of myself, I promise I will move back home."

She agreed...six months later.

I had to convince my mom that I would be responsible enough to go to LA for school once I got there. Every day, when my mom came home from work, I would have printouts of information on every community college, including all the details of how to attend and the transfer process. I included every apartment complex or student housing that I could find, and we would go over them together. It was my daily report to her to let her know how serious I was about this move. My mom's coworker was also a parent of a young adult with a disability, and she gave my mom tips about what she had to do to gain confidence in me. Once my mom felt that I was capable enough to live independently, her coworker got her to agree officially. As we began putting into place the details of how we were going to make this work, my sister volunteered to come to LA as my caregiver. Naturally, this made my mom even more sure that we were making the right decision.

We found a place, completed the transfer process to the community college, and we all headed to Los Angeles. My sister and I were moving into an apartment we had never toured in person, and what we got was a tiny apartment with brick walls, one bedroom, one bathroom with the shower and toilet in one room, and the sink in the bedroom area. The shower was so old that no matter how much bleach you put on it, some stains would not lift. I was still incredibly grateful because all I wanted to do was move to LA and keep going after that dream; and I was finally here.

I knew that the decision to leave my comfort zone so I could make my dream a reality was necessary. Choosing to move to LA with no real plan and just a gut feeling was, to this day, the best decision I've made in my life. It was because of the decisions I made as a teenager that I was able to create a life that is different from what anyone would've ever expected, especially the doctors and their numbers. It shocks me every time I think back on it. "Like, damn girl, you had some real nerve." It was way more than that, though. Unbeknownst to me, this simple yet powerful decision would be the beginning of how I made all of my most critical life decisions moving forward. It's a mixture of following my gut (which I like to call God's way of speaking to me) and unwavering faith. I have this muscle because of my mom. I was able to strengthen it because of what my mom introduced me to once I moved to Los Angeles. It's my favorite natural law, the Law of Attraction.

> **Side note:** That conversation was over sixteen years ago. I haven't moved back to Stockton since. You'll learn later how LA was whooping my ass, figuratively speaking, but I've truly made it my home.

Roll It Back

Fighting to get out of a comfort zone is the result of a dream goal you have that has been nagging at you and your gut to accomplish. The dream doesn't have to involve such a big, life-changing decision as I had to make. It could be about getting a dream car, new apartment, new job, new relationship, dream vacation destination—whatever it is that is making you realize that you may be stagnant, yet you feel an urgency to push to new heights. This is the feeling to follow to get out of that comfort zone. It's hard! It's scary! And there's no guarantee that pushing out of your comfort zone is going to keep you "comfortable" as you grow. Although growing isn't comfortable, it is always worth it. Regardless of outside people doubting your capabilities or you doubting yourself, the thing that is guaranteed is that as you grow, you will get better.

Get Rolling

Recognize You're in a Comfort Zone

Being in a comfort zone is not a bad thing. Many people are completely happy with where their lives are and enjoy a sense of safety. That's beautiful. But for those who are still wanting more from life experiences and opportunities, we need to recognize the signs that we're stuck in a comfort zone and need to push ourselves to the next level of achievements. Here are some signs to reflect on to help recognize if you're stuck in a comfort zone.

1. **Are there any productive habits you've stopped doing?** My grades slipping in college was a major shock that my behaviors were changing for the worse—one of the biggest signs that I was in a comfort zone. Other examples would be, for someone who may have a fitness goal—did you stop going to the gym? Did you stop meal-prepping? Or in general, are you not journaling? Not reading? Not spending time on your hobbies? Anything along those lines should push you to see how you can get back to those habits.

2. **Do you feel more excited, or more stagnant, on a regular basis?** It's okay to have days that are more routine, but how do you *feel* during your daily routines? When I was skipping classes, it was because I wanted to have a reason to feel more excited and alive in what I

was doing. Going to my classes felt mundane because
I wasn't being challenged to achieve anything new or
bigger than what I already knew.

3. **Is it time to change your environment?** I believe
   people don't pay attention enough to the impact their
   environments have on their overall well-being. Your
   environment—whether it be your cubicle at work, your
   home, or the city you live in—affects the rate at which you
   grow into our best self. Because I stayed in Stockton after
   high school, I was still around the same people I'd spent
   every day with for the previous four years, and lived in the
   same bedroom I had been in since middle school, there
   was nothing that felt like it was changing for the better.
   Sure, I was an "adult," but I was still living the same lifestyle
   as a teenager. And if nothing was changing around me,
   then how could I think something would change out of
   nowhere without action? I had to make a move.

Break Out of Your Comfort Zone

Although in many ways a comfort zone sounds like a good
idea because it keeps you safe from your insecurities and
unforeseen pain or traumas, it is detrimental to your growth.
If I had chosen to stay in Stockton because I had built a
foundation where I could stay safe at home with my mom, I
would not be able to have the successful independent life I live
today. Hell, I wouldn't be able to have anything to share in this
book with you.

Here's what I suggest you can do to work toward making
the decision to break out of your comfort zone:

1. **Get excited about the possibilities of achieving your dream.** We all have the dream life we desire, big or small, but regardless of how you size it up, if it gets you excited, then it's worth going after. Research other people who are living that dream and learn their stories as proof that it's possible. Research anything relevant to making your dream possible. Whether it's classes, apartments, cars, careers, or anything else, you have to get it out of your head and into your hands to start building your dream with real-life information. You always have a reference for what could be achieved next, so you don't stay stuck.

2. **Don't sweat the plan.** The plan for having it all figured out doesn't need to be perfect. Have you ever made plans to do something you wanted, and everything worked out perfectly? Have you ever worked out how to do something you wanted, and it went all wrong? If you answered yes to both and you're reading this book, then that means you made it through both times. So no matter how much you do or don't plan, no matter how things turn out, you know you will make it through. Stop delaying to make the perfect plan and start moving even if you don't have one.

3. **Your gut feeling is *very* real.** We all have intuition, and your gut is just a manifestation of that. It's a natural law to "sense" something, even if it's not in front of you or hasn't happened yet. With your dreams, it's the same sense that will bug you until you make a decision. We all have dreams, but there's a reason your dreams are recurring; they are meant for you to achieve.

Chapter 4

I-N-D-E-P-E-N-D-E-N-T

"There was something about knowing that I was taking care of my responsibilities on my own that warranted a sense of pride and maturity that allowed me to start exercising the freedoms of going out and partying."

The Law of Attraction is a natural law that works like the spiritual concept of karma—whatever you put out into the universe is what you'll get back. When people reference this law, it is traditionally used as a positivity exercise to help people change their lives for the better. There are multiple exercises that activate the law, like vision boarding, journaling, meditation etc.

Looking back, I recognize that I had been using the law during my high school years without even knowing that it existed (i.e., not accepting that AOL search as my future). But when I first intentionally started implementing the law in my life, it was through positive thinking, affirmations, and good ol' faith once I moved to Los Angeles. The combination of these is what laid the foundation to keep me motivated to stay in the city through the toughest times.

Living in Los Angeles on my own was a dream come true. The excitement I felt to take on the world after first moving was overwhelming at times, but always in a good way. Remember earlier, when I described how I knew I needed to move to LA to live my life but had no real plans? Well, I learned very

quickly how unprepared I actually was to navigate the city
with a disability. You also must keep in mind that, at that point,
I was still fresh to using the electric wheelchair. Adjusting
to new ways of life was flying at me all at once and it was up
to me to figure it out. I wasn't in Stockton anymore with the
security blanket of my mom, friends, and high school; I was in
the big leagues.

The first lesson in my independence was navigating
public transportation. I did not have the ability physically or
financially to drive, so I had to figure out ways to get from my
530-square-foot apartment to the community college that was
a twenty-minute driving distance away. I first tried the local
disability door-to-door transportation service, Dial-A-Ride.
This was essentially what Uber and Lyft are now, but it was only
for people with disabilities. The only differences are that you
don't get to request on-demand, and you share the ride with
multiple people who get dropped off along the way to your
route. You must allow the vans a four-hour window to pick
you up, and if they can't find you, they will leave you without
notice—only for you to realize, after you've been waiting for an
hour *past* the designated four-hour window, that the driver
left you and you have to find another way home. If I needed
to be on campus by 10:00 a.m. to make it to my first class, I
had to allow the drivers to show up anytime between 6:00
and 10:00 a.m. to pick me up. Which means technically I had
to be ready to go by 6:00 a.m., because if the driver decided
to come get me at 6:15 and I wasn't ready, I would be left to
scramble on how to get to school without them. Then, if I was
ready by 6:15 and they had just a couple more pickups on the
way to my destination, arriving by 8:00, I'd have to wait around
on campus until 10:00 before my first class began. This was
the reality of my independence for the first few months. It was
incredibly stressful for me, and showed a huge hole in how the

lives of people with disabilities were valued. I knew I couldn't keep going back and forth to school like this, especially after crying to my mom on multiple days after the drivers had consistently left me. I needed to find another way, because moving back to Stockton was not an option. My next option was public transportation, a.k.a. the city bus. I had to learn the bus routes fast because I was fed up with a service that claimed it was designed to help people with disabilities.

The Bus. Talk about a journey. To get from my apartment to my campus, I had to ride my wheelchair through the university that was across the street and up one block to my first bus stop; take that bus for thirty minutes to my next bus; take my second bus another thirty minutes to my college campus stop; and then ride two blocks in my wheelchair and through an empty field to get onto the campus where my classes were. That ride would take a total of two hours each way on any given day, five days a week, for two years. This was the start to a series of experiences in my life that started my grind toward achieving my dreams. I look back on these years and remember how determined I felt not to let anything get in the way of making the life I desired happen. If the bus was my best option to go to school and live in LA, then that's what I was going to do.

Because everything was new for me, I took on all-new experiences with the best attitude I could, even when I made the big decision to change my major from my childhood dream of journalism to a newfound passion for video editing. Making this decision was a major lesson for me in how deciding to change your game plan on the journey toward your dreams can really make a difference in the outcome of your future. Having a successful career in journalism was the reason I'd decided to move to LA, but once I was here, I was struck with a new passion I didn't expect to have. I took a course on video journalism, where video editing was part of completing the semester's assignment, and I fell in love. I knew that it was time to make the shift, change directions in my higher education, and focus on this new passion.

When you're on your journey to achieving your dreams, circumstances regularly change, and our decision-making skills are put to the test. But time, experience, and even new environments present opportunities to discover new and unexpected things about yourself. Most importantly, I had to prove to myself that I could make this dream a reality. When we set goals to achieve our dreams, we have to know that it'll take work, and that that's the part we can't avoid. No matter how advanced technology gets, or how much social media continues to take over our lives, the grind to attain success is inevitable. In order to stay on the grind, you need whatever motivation you can get to help you overcome any speed bumps along the way. The fact that I had wanted to move to LA for a life of success convinced my mom that I could handle living independently. The constant reminder that I needed to prove AOL's prediction about my future wrong was the fuel I needed to wake up in the morning and get on that bus every day. The best way to stay focused, once you decide on your motivation, is concentrating on each smaller goal, one at a time. Thinking of the bigger dream can feel overwhelming. We can get lost in our self-pressured expectation of what we should or shouldn't have achieved within a certain amount of time. My focus was to get through community college with my associate degree to finally transfer to the university I lived across the street from. And I did.

When I began living across the street from my university, I still had to use the bus to go *everywhere* else. From doctors' appointments to shopping malls to work, I was on the bus. And that was my only way of getting around independently for the next twelve years after that. Taking the bus while living in LA was never part of my plan. I had a perception of what I thought living in LA could look like, but you never really know until you're already deep into making the dream happen. I don't know if there is such a thing as being prepared enough. You can only prepare with as much knowledge as you have at the moment when planning to achieve something that you desire. Life experience is the greatest teacher, and the unexpected moments or sudden challenges are what help grow you into a person who, more than likely, you never knew you could turn out to be. But learning how to pivot in those moments will be the key you need to continue to handle those unexpected changes along your journey. With each challenge conquered, the stronger the steel you have to fight for what's yours. Had I treated taking the bus as a be-all-end-all situation (because it was never part of my plan) and used it as a reason to go back to Stockton and give up on everything, I know I would not be where I'm at today. You can't let the unexpected make you feel like you are not ready for your dreams or push you back into your comfort zone.

I officially stopped using the bus as the main means of transportation when I quit my job at the top of 2020. During my time using the bus, I had been harassed, annoyed, and bothered on multiple occasions. But my determination to make something of myself was still too strong to give up; however, I knew I needed more support before this whole experience became too overwhelming. When you're faced with minimal options in life, you have to take what's given to you and make it work. This is the root of creativity and innovation when you are, like I was, someone who doesn't have any resources available to create opportunities. Luckily the internet has grown to be a resource with an infinite amount of information, where you can research something you don't have much knowledge about when working to move on to the next stage in your journey toward the dream. Learning the stories of currently successful people, taking online classes, or finding creditable influencers can all be game-changing resources. During these times of exploration and creativity, I realized the foundation that I created and was afforded in high school was something I was going to have to build from the ground up again. Having the support of others is crucial to a person's success. And, although I realized how much I missed having my friends and family near me, I still knew that going back to Stockton was not an option. Instead, I decided that it was time to put myself out there to make a new foundation of friends that would turn into the family I needed if I planned on staying in LA. Knowing this, I would use the Law of Attraction again to put out the energy that I wanted to make friends.

It wasn't until I started making friends at college that turned everything around for me. It all started when I befriended the first girl I met in the off-campus dorm that I moved into. I borrowed a DVD (yes, it was still DVD days) and, when I went to her place to drop it off, I met friends she was already hanging out with—and everything grew from there. We became friends quickly and are still very close to this day. The special bond that I continued to build with new people from around my building was centered at my apartment. My place was the spot everyone went to hang out. This then turned into the spot everyone partied at on the weekends, since many of us were still too young to go to clubs in Hollywood. It was the best communal experience I've ever had. We studied together, did each other's nails, and my cousin (RIP), who was a barber, would cut everyone's hair. We had movie nights too, and when we did become old enough to go to the club, my place was the pregame spot before we all went out together to turn up for the rest of the night. So many people were in and out of my place that I used to just keep my door unlocked.

College set a different tone for me than high school. There was something about knowing that I was taking care of my responsibilities on my own that warranted a sense of pride and maturity that allowed me to start exercising the freedoms of going out and partying. The foundation of friends that I had made so far were all more supportive in unexpected ways, and I knew I could trust them to be sure I was always okay, even without my mom around. Sometimes staying in your comfort zone prevents you from taking risks, and, since I had successfully taken the risk to move to LA, I knew I could handle having a social life too. In order to make friends, I had to be part of the social scene. This group wasn't doing anything that made me feel unsafe or uncomfortable, so I was more willing to take risks than I had been in high school. And because we were all college students, we had something important to lose, so we never took our risk-taking too far. We stayed near places we knew would be safe while allowing ourselves the freedom to have a good time. I was so comfortable that it was like having the same foundation of family and friends as I had during high school, but this time on a more elevated level.

Because I was clear on the other side of California and in college, I was learning adulthood through every experience. I was in constant decision-making mode. Like, "Should I go to class, or sleep in because I'm exhausted from finals week?" or "Should I spend this last $10 on food, or on my bus fare for the week?"

Every day was a learning experience set off by actions that came with reactions. Just like in high school, my college friends loved me for exactly who I was. Nothing felt weird or different—which, I can't lie, I was nervous about at first, because these people didn't know me the way the friends

I had grown up with knew me. These people met me as a person with a disability, and every time I showed I could ambulate, it was like they'd witnessed a Jesus-level miracle happening right in front of them. That is, until I explained my disability further, and then it would be on to the next topic of conversation. I felt less alone in needing to figure everything out on my own now. We bonded so much, we literally became a crew.

One of my favorite memories is of a time when we were all sitting around starving, but none of us had enough money that we could pool it together and buy enough food for all of us to eat. What we did instead was take whatever leftovers we each had, put them together, and create a potluck for each other. We literally went from room to room with our plates and grabbed a little bit of each other's food in each room, and by the time we were done, we all had a full-fledged meal together. Moments like these are a reminder of the importance of having a foundation of support for your life as you work toward your successes. The power of networking is that you find like-minded people who have the same goals and beliefs as you do—including people who are talented in ways you are not—your intentions can come together, and you can collaborate on a specific goal, hoping to inspire others. You need to have your network to build toward your dreams because it is impossible to do it all by yourself. A team is needed to delegate tasks to, even if you're not in position to build a full team yet. You are much more powerful linking and building communities of people with different talents and skills to create with a common intention to share talents with the world.

My college friends are such a special group; they took on the unspoken responsibility of making sure I was always taken care of and included in anything we did. They became equally creative and demanding of accessibility for me as we navigated parties, clubs, group outings—literally, for anything we planned as a group, they considered whether I would be able to go too and would find solutions if, for whatever reason, accessibility was an issue. These are the people you need to have in your life. Disability or not, having a solid foundation of friends who consider you and your needs before making any decisions is necessary to building a successful life. It's a special bond to grow into adulthood with a group of equally wide-eyed young people you've met while in college. It's an experience I will never forget.

This group of people is the cornerstone of how successful you will be. Will Smith once said, "You are only as successful as the five closest people to you," and I feel that entirely. If I hadn't had such an amazing group of people around me during that time, who genuinely loved me as I am, I don't think I would've been successful at staying in LA. This makes me think back on how crucial this specific time of my life was to ultimately fulfilling my purpose. I needed to master life as independently as possible in order to know that I had the life skills to keep pushing toward my dream, which at the time was to be a renowned, well-respected video editor. But the next phase I entered would be like nothing I had ever experienced before.

Roll It Back

Taking a leap of faith is never simple, so stop trying to find the "easy" way to do it. The reason a leap is invigorating is that we know the challenges of trying something new and the uncertainty of it working out in our favor. Preparation is good, so long as you use it as a tool to grow versus as an excuse to not make a move forward. Preparing allows us to create some level of comfort in taking a risk, but you'll never be prepared enough for the unexpected. Accepting that there's only so much you can do to prepare for a risk before fully leaning into faith will make your decision-making a much more doable process. Opening yourself up to new experiences will help you continue to develop tools to better your judgment as you make decisions toward the desires of your heart. New experiences allow for unpredictable outcomes, but that's what makes the journey a wonderful story to tell in the future. Because, at the end of the day, taking the opportunity to go after your dreams, regardless of which experiences cause you to pivot or change, is always beneficial to your growth as a human being. Growing to become a better version of yourself creates those opportunities to meet like-minded people, which in turn allows you to be fed by others' energies. This will help propel you into more varied and new experiences and present chances to explore more on your journey to your dreams.

Get Rolling

Decide to Grind

When working toward any goal, you must prepare to grind hard and pivot. Putting in the work is inevitable, and there's no cheat code or faster way to get there. Even if you're one of the few who get to their goal quickly, you still have to work to maintain the success and continue to grow from there. Here are some tips to help keep you on your grind:

1. **Understand your "why."** Why are you wanting to reach a particular goal? What is motivating you to do so? And

why now? My goal of not returning to Stockton because I wanted more for my life was one reason. Wanting to see how fruitful a life I could create for myself despite having a disability was another. Both were strong enough for me to not give up.

2. **Get used to the pivot.** Unexpected changes are never fun for anyone; however, if you can master how to pivot with positivity, the changes will become less and less startling every time. My switching from using Dial-A-Ride to taking the bus on my own is one of many pivots I had to make on my journey toward my dream. Pivoting is a skill every person should really grasp how to do, especially once you realize that life is just one ever-changing cycle.

3. **Focus on one small goal at a time.** Doing this will keep you more focused and confident as you continue to go after your dreams. When we think about the end goal and all of the steps it takes to get there, it can quickly become overwhelming. A major goal is never meant to be completed in a short period of time. There's a reason that, in sports, an entire season of games has to be played, with numerous practices between them, before a team is even considered to play in a championship. You must conquer the workout, then the practice, then the game on repeat for months, before you get to the playoffs, then the championship game. In the words of my greatest distant mentor Nipsey Hussle, "It's a marathon."

Decide on Your Foundation

Creating your own foundation or team of supportive people is as imperative for your health as it is for your successes. The company we keep matters because the influences of those closest to us energetically affect our decisions. You want to surround yourself with people who have the same morals and goals you do, although they should have different skillsets that support achieving a goal for everyone involved.

When choosing who you spend time with, you can ask yourself the following questions:

1. Does this person have a big dream they're passionately working toward?

2. Does this person have a skillset that I don't, and vice versa? Can we support each other's goals using our different talents?

3. Do you think this person is good at making strong decisions? Do they factor the pros and cons? Are they open to multiple ways of finding a solution?

Chapter 5

THIS SOME BULLSH*T

"I knew I was harming myself by living like this, but I couldn't get myself to want to leave LA."

Society tells us that to be successful you have to go to school, get good grades, go to college, and get a degree, so that you'll be able to find a job immediately, because this degree weeds you out from everyone else. While this may be true in some industries and professions, it did not quite go the same way for me as a college graduate with a degree in TV production. However, because my degree was in a more creative field, I did get the freedom to decide to work for myself as a freelance video editor.

Since I was fresh from graduating college and everyone in my LA foundation had all gone their separate ways for various reasons, I was back on a different grind. It was more serious for me now because, just like in high school, I had to figure out this next stage in life, but this time with absolutely no school staff to keep me safe. I had entered real adulthood. I had to move out of my off-campus dorm and decided to get into my own apartment—this time without roommates, completely solo for the first time. I found a studio apartment in, not the worst neighborhood, but certainly not the best. It was only 530 square feet, but it was all mine. Rent was $950 and, since I was no longer receiving the assistance of student loans, the only income I had was SSI (Supplemental Security Income), which was $750 a month. Mind you, I still had to pay utilities, food, household, and recreation expenses after making up for the $200 shortfall between SSI and rent. Saving money for the future or emergencies was not even an option.

This is the reality of most people living with disabilities who have to rely on government assistance to live independently. SSI is a government program that pays disabled and elderly people monthly benefits for their living expenses. When I was on SSI in 2012, the maximum amount of monthly support was $750. Fast-forward over ten years later, and the maximum amount is now $841, a $91 difference…yeah, some bullshit. The amount of income you receive is not based on location, either. For me, living in Los Angeles, which was back then and still is one of the most expensive cities to live in in the United States, the 2012 maximum amount of $750 got me virtually nowhere because the cost of living there was always going to force me to live beyond my means so long as I had to rely on SSI for income. If you decide to get a job as a person with a disability on SSI, unless the job pays triple the SSI amount, finding employment is not worth doing. Because, if the job only pays even a little over your monthly SSI amount, the government will stop your benefits. And if somehow you are lucky enough to have more than $2,000 in your bank account at any given time, throughout any month, while on SSI, you will be completely removed from the program, forcing you through the long and tedious process of reapplying later, should you need it. And there's still no guarantee that you'll be able to qualify again. And, if you're on SSI, there is no other form of government assistance that you are able to qualify for either. It's SSI only.

These very real circumstances are telltale signs of how much the government truly does not want to help or support the disabled community, and how it keeps a vicious cycle of dependency going for people with disabilities. It makes the

option of exploring your dreams, or even simply exploring
the best versions of yourself, difficult and rare, rather than
part of the natural progression of life as it is for anyone else.
There's a lot you can learn about the world and yourself when
you're disabled and living independently, but the chances of
us getting those opportunities are slim—because the upkeep,
depending on your disability, can cost you upwards of $5,000
a month in medical expenses alone, in addition to the living
expenses of an average independent adult. I can tell you,
$750 a month doesn't even scratch the surface of what it costs
a person with a disability to live independently. So when I
made the choice to continue to live in LA after graduating
college to live solely on my SSI, I knew I was up against
the impossible.

Knowing I had to make a living for myself, I had to come
up with a game plan. It was either that or move back, and
I would be damned if I had come this far just to have to go
back. Asking for money from my family had to be a last-
resort option, only under dire circumstances, because my
family didn't have much to spare either, nor did I want them
panicking, thinking that something was wrong in LA. They
would then try to convince me to leave. I was on my own for
this one. With my degree in TV production (with an emphasis
in video editing), I started by tapping into the network of
people I'd befriended while at college. These people were
directors and producers; I let them know I was available to
work and to edit any content they might be working on.

Throughout college, my sister and I had created a series of
mock music videos, where we took a mainstream artist's song
and filmed a music video version of it to post online. These
were really thought-out video narratives, quality content,
that gained a lot of attention and popularity at the time. We
even did one for the song "Killers" by Drake, featuring Nipsey

Hussle, and Nipsey retweeted the link. That was one of the most exciting days of my life, because what my love for Nipsey and his music did for me at this time would be completely life-changing later. But we'll get back to that. Because of the popularity of those videos, when my other creative friends found out I was freelance editing full time, some paid me to do some work for them. This is why I emphasized in previous chapters the importance of building a foundation and a network. In those times when you need support in a significant way, there will be people there who are willing to step up. Having a network is like building your own community of people rooted in the same values as you—people with varied talents, different from your own, so you can tap into each other's gifts to build something great.

The challenge of living as a freelancer in any creative skill is that money isn't consistent. You can't guarantee when your next job will come in. And since social media wasn't nearly as powerful then as it is today, the grind felt twice as hard as it had in college. Before, my grind was a bit more standard. I just had to learn how to navigate LA on my own. But I had school and friends to support my other basic needs, so I didn't feel as if I was left out in the cold. But now I was grinding to eat, keep a roof over my head, keep my heat and electricity on, build a successful career so that I would not fail and have to go back home; I was grinding to stay alive. Any little bit of additional income helped.

I was editing promo videos that my friend was producing for a university, I did music videos for up-and-coming local artists with tiny budgets, and I did behind-the-scenes videos of music video production for mainstream artists. The big lesson I learned was that, even though I was strapped for cash during this time, barely scraping by, I was never too prideful to still do some work for free. What I learned quickly was that, sometimes, having a credit attached to a major celebrity or major project would be more valuable than having the money itself. This is the backward, smoke-and-mirrors side of the entertainment industry. The smaller organizations or artists with tiny budgets were keeping me paid and staying in LA, but the projects with bigger names were almost never paid. When the projects with major people involved were made public, others who knew nothing about the business would see it and think I was living large; as a result, other creatives, usually without a lot of money, or with content I simply didn't want to work on, would see these credits and want to hire me. Meanwhile, I was having to choose between getting to eat or to keep my electricity on. My reality was saying yes to every project, no matter how much the check was, just so I could have a little bit more to get me to the next day.

This was one of the toughest times I had experienced living in LA up to this point, because I was playing with sacrificing my health for my dream—all because of the unhealthy drive to prove that AOL search wrong yet again. When a non-disabled person chooses to make everyday sacrifices in exchange for staying steadfast on their grind, the same options are not available to a person with a disability. Non-disabled people in the same position would probably be able to rent a room out of a random person's house, have a ton of roommates or, hell, live in their car to save on rent costs—not folks with disabilities. Physical safety is paramount to all our needs, and we can't risk that in the same way that others can. Some non-disabled people may be able to work two to three odd jobs, then work on their passions afterwards—not people with disabilities. Employment for people with disabilities is not easy to come by, let alone the transportation to get to each job. And lack of sleep can quickly become detrimental to our physical health. Non-disabled people may even risk their freedom by having illegal or immoral hustles, no judgment at all, but—not people with disabilities. Doing anything illegal is not an option, because surviving in prison is too wild to even have to fathom for a person with a disability. Living with myself and my own mental health is just as important as—if not more important than—my physical health at times. I was offered many opportunities for money that I know would've changed everything around for me—at the sacrifice of my morals—including adult entertainment, but I decided not to. I'll be honest—I thought about it, but still decided against it. That's how tough it was for me during that time.

When life gets that tough, your morals, health, and mental well-being all get tested at the same time. The lines you thought you could draw and the boundaries you thought you could hold start to blur and crumble. I wasn't eating. I wasn't sleeping. I was constantly trying to figure out ways to make money while keeping a smile on my face and telling my family and friends back home that everything was fine— until I couldn't take it anymore. The last bit of fight I had in me folded, and I broke down one day. I was in my apartment crying until my head and eyes hurt. I was screaming into my pillow out of frustration and fear. I knew I was harming myself by living like this, but I couldn't get myself to want to leave LA. I didn't know what to do, but I knew I had to do something and do it fast. Whatever decision I had to make next was going to be the make-or-break for me staying in LA.

I took the next few days to relax, because I was mentally and emotionally exhausted, and then my dad introduced me to the book *The Alchemist*. This book changed my life. It's about a young boy, Santiago, who goes on a journey to chase his dream of finding an extravagant treasure, and along the way, runs into various people and has unique experiences and challenges that ultimately all play into his ability to reach his goal. The book resonated with me so much that it felt almost like an extension of everything I had trained myself to do as I was mastering the Law of Attraction. It was what I needed to see to know that I was on the right path. At the time, I relied a lot on the music of Nipsey Hussle as well. The music he was putting out then was speaking to my experience of being on the grind toward a dream, to a tee. A common theme in his music is his slogan, "The Marathon." Listening to his songs was a constant reminder that chasing the dream is a marathon, not a sprint.

Life is going to test you. People are going to test you. Society is going to test you, but you have to keep going. God got you. Utilizing what I was learning through the power of storytelling and music was the tipping point toward the right direction for what I needed to keep going. Having these various art forms, or just external outlets, to help give you confidence in what you're trying to accomplish is necessary to help you push through those gut-wrenching times. There's only so much a person can handle on their own, so we must seek those tools that are separate from us or our loved ones to help keep us focused. Sometimes we think making a decision is solely rooted in proactively thinking about the next big move, or the next best move to avoid failure, when really the next best decision might be to sit still. Cry it out. Give yourself some grace that you are human and, as long as you are trying, that is enough progress for the universe to recognize your greatness and continue to bless you on your journey.

Roll It Back

This is the part of adulthood they don't prepare you for at any level of education, which can throw you into straight survival mode as soon as you leave the nest of "school." The catch-22 in living under survival circumstances is that, in the moment when these experiences are happening, they feel (and in many ways are) some of the worst you could ever have. But when you navigate through to the other side of your worst days, the solutions you find for yourself are invaluable to your growth moving forward. The wild thing is that you will continue to go through difficult challenges, and, because you have already made it through one situation, you'll know how to get through the next much more easily.

In many ways, some of those solutions may not be the proudest moment of your life, but it's something we should never be ashamed of when our intentions are pure. That's why I believe having a positive support group of family or friends helps you stay on track with doing the right things as much as possible. Their outside perspectives can help you with creative solutions during tough times. The support system of others assists us in seeing outside the box because, when those moral boundaries start to blur, they help you refocus and see clearly. Tough times are inevitable, and no matter how hard we try to avoid them, it's impossible. We can feel like we are preparing for anticipated failures, but we never know how these experiences are going to show up, or what they're meant to teach us. The only way to get through them is to brace yourself for the ride.

Get Rolling

Decisions Can Be Harmful. Be Careful!

When you are in a constant state of needing to prove something to others and to yourself, that determination can push you into some potentially rocky territory at times. We must, no matter how badly we want something, be able to recognize the signs that we are probably taking the grind too far. I'm sharing these tips to help you avoid the consequences of some of my potentially dangerous decisions in an effort to support your journey.

1. **If you must lie about your well-being to your loved ones, reevaluate.** Any healthy positive relationships you have with others should never make you want to lie to them. We only do this when we know we are doing something harmful to ourselves that they wouldn't approve of. Depend on loved ones for support, instead avoiding them out of fear that they may hold a mirror to your face and make you look at yourself.

2. **Sacrifices are normal, but not if you are starving.** I know we live in a toxic hustle culture, where we are told that if we are not pushing ourselves to our complete breaking points, we are not trying hard enough. I like to challenge that by putting a different perspective on that message. Yes, sacrifice is part of the process; yes, we must push past our comfort zones; yes, we must challenge ourselves to do new things. But there is nothing great about the grind if your mind and body are not functioning at a healthy capacity. Keep your mental and physical health the ultimate priority, and everything else will fall into place.

3. **Your network is your next check.** As you already know, networking and building your foundation creates the necessary support system for when you need to make decisions. If it weren't for tapping into those fellow creatives to ask for help and lending my talent as

support to their work, I wouldn't have made it—I'd be back home. That's what your network is for, and when it's your turn to support back, do it and do it graciously.

External Tools Can Be Your Lifesaver or Life-Changer

When reviewing the tools for what it takes to be successful, we can sometimes overlook the smaller things that help us get through each day. But, as I mentioned before with *The Alchemist* and Nipsey Hussle, books, music, art, podcasts, videos, etc., can all be resources to help you boost your confidence and drive when nothing else is giving you wind under your wings. Here are ways to determine which external tools to consider for your journey.

1. **What makes your spirit light up?** Pay close attention to when you laugh and smile, recognize the cause of it, and use those things whenever you can to have a moment to smile each day.

2. **Does this tool help you or distract you from your grind?** I know distractions usually aren't revered as helpful when on a mission, but I like to believe a healthy form of distraction is helpful. Maybe think of those things you like that have *nothing* to do with your work. Or consider tools that are new and completely different from your work. These can provide moments of clarity at the most-needed times if you let them.

3. **Can this tool help you in other ways outside of your dream chase?** Not every tool you'll learn from has to do with the grind itself. Sometimes these tools are there to

help you become better in other areas of your life that
can then positively affect your journey.

Chapter 6
BUT WHAT ABOUT RENT?

"This was true independence for someone like me."

Now, don't get it twisted; the struggle was still so very real. Although I had found the external tools to get my spirit and hopes back up, the challenges were still there. At least now I could think a bit more clearly about what I was doing; I could focus on my next decision to keep going. This is the time when I had to get very real about what I was putting myself through to achieve this dream and stay in Los Angeles. I looked around at my life. I was grateful that I had magically been able to maintain rent and utilities for my place. I still had clothes to get me through my days, thanks to hand-me-downs from my friends. I used to tell them I liked thrift clothes so they would bring stuff they outgrew when, really, I could never buy anything new. Then I took a deeper look, and knew I wasn't taking care of my physical health. I remember a friend telling me at that time, "You can't live out your dream if your body shuts down." And my response was, "True, but all I need is just enough work to get by and, once I have the money, I can hire a chef to cook for me and never have to worry about food again." Yeah—that's how delusionally determined I was. And when I was having this honest conversation with myself, I recognized that I was pushing my disabled body in a direction that was not good. I wasn't eating three meals a day. Sometimes I could only afford to eat once a day, and would have a snack and go to bed early so I wouldn't get hungry again and have to come up with a meal for dinner; I knew I didn't have enough to eat. When I did have food, I had to make it stretch. My food usually consisted of a mix of fried bologna sandwiches, Vienna sausages and rice, cans of chili, packs of ramen noodles, and—when I wanted to get fancy because it had been a good-paying freelance week— tilapia tostadas. I am grateful for those meals that helped get me by, but none of that is healthy for any person to eat on a regular basis, let alone a person with a disability whose physical well-being is rooted in healthy eating. I was twenty-seven years old and weighed ninety-five pounds. Yeah, something had to give.

This brutally honest self-reflection part is what most people like to skip through or avoid. Not many people, in the midst of their struggle, have the courage to admit to themselves that their lives are failing and failing fast, and then also admit that *they* are the ones who did it to themselves. It wasn't an easy conversation with myself, but I was all tapped out on trying to do it alone and thinking I had all the answers. I needed help. At a certain point, we must face what is real and not be so focused on our futures that we are destroying ourselves in the process. The only answer I could find was making the decision to get a traditional paying job. This was another pivot decision I had to make. It is okay to have a traditional job while working toward your bigger dream. I know the toxic hustle culture in entertainment, specifically, will have you believe you can't work because you have to be available for auditions, or be available every time you get a gig. Or you can't get a job because it takes away the focus from plan A, and that's the only plan that should consume your mind. But having a job can still be part of plan A, with the understanding that whatever is for you will be for you. Your priority has to be working a job first, because you need to keep a roof over your head and, in my case, literally become physically healthier.

Whatever gig you miss out on because of your job, just know that it wasn't meant for you and that's okay. The right job for you will come, and the universe will provide a way to make it available for you to be part of. And I have plenty of proof of that to share with you in future chapters. It is possible to do both. You've just got to find your balance, but it's by no means "working backward" to have a traditional job while working toward your dreams.

Remember, I was still on SSI, so technically this was not something I was supposed to be doing, but I felt I had no other choice. I started job hunting. I figured if I got a low-enough-paying job that it wouldn't flag SSI, and with the money I got from that small job, I'd have just enough to cover my living expenses. I searched far and wide on the internet for jobs that I could do. When you have a disability and use a mobility device like a wheelchair, there are a multitude of things you have to consider before you can even apply for a job.

- Is the location of the interview and job accessible?
- Does the position require any heavy physical lifting?
- Do the company staff seem like nice enough people to even want to hire a person with a disability?
- Would I need any desk accommodations? (I hate to even have to ask.)
- Can I get to and from the job on the bus?

All of these questions were necessary because, at that time, working from home was not an option (LOL, the world changes all of a sudden when everyone has to experience disability. #COVID).

And those were just the things to think about regarding my disability. I still had to qualify through level of education, the proper degree, number of years of experience, and computer program skillsets, on top of everything else. After months of searching, I landed a part-time, minimum-wage-plus-commission job at a call center, recycling cell phones. Was this job ideal? Absolutely not, but it was the only company, after months of submitting my résumé and going on interviews, that actually hired me. It was in this janky office space, with side-by-side cubicles, and the employees were the most diverse group of people I'd ever seen. Of course, the supervisor tried to encourage us by sharing the types of bonuses we could get if we applied ourselves and nailed the script. We would randomly call various businesses and ask them if they had any cell phones they needed to recycle and, if so, we'd send them a shipping label to have them shipped to our offices to be recycled. Based on how many cell phones we were able to collect from businesses, that would determine what our bonuses would be. I didn't get many bonuses, nor did I really care.

Doing a job where 80 percent of what you do involves false leads, no answers, or people either hanging up on you or cursing you out was not good for my mental or emotional health. I was just trying to get my weekly paycheck so I could mix that with the freelance work I was still getting, just to have enough to keep getting by. But because I told myself that my health now had to come before my dream (which you would think is an obvious standard to set for yourself, but it definitely wasn't for me), I had to quit my call center job. It was negatively affecting me, and the one-hour round-trip bus ride to get there every day was feeling more like a drag than a gratitude. But since I knew I was quitting, I knew I had to find my next job quickly to supplement with that extra income *again*, or else it was all bad for me.

This is why it's important to fully understand your boundaries when working toward your goals. Many times, when we discuss boundaries, it is in reference to other people or outside forces. For me, I believe we need to also set boundaries within ourselves, to be sure we don't push beyond our own limits and end up in an unhealthy place. We have to know what our stopping points are, so we know when it's time to safely remove ourselves from a situation. Quitting a job is never easy. The best way to gauge when it's time to quit something and move on to the next thing is to pay attention to how it's affecting your mind, body, and spirit. If you are being impacted negatively, it's time to let go and move on. If there isn't much affecting you directly, and you simply don't like something because it's not easy, you may want to reconsider your decision. Sacrificing your time for the job because of the big-picture priorities it supports, while managing your off time so you can work on what you love, is sometimes needed.

Once I quit the call center job, it was time to pivot again. This time, I focused my job hunt on opportunities that were part of the entertainment industry, because I knew that's where I had the most experience. This took another two months of interviews and résumé sending before I landed an internship with a movie distribution company in their marketing department. The work was not in video editing as I had hoped. I knew it would be tedious (and presumably unpaid, because it was an internship). But to be working for a credited company in the industry that specialized in all things having to do with Black films, I knew the value of working there at any capacity was greater than money itself. I knew I nailed my first interview because of my inherent knowledge of Black films combined with the skills I'd learned in college. I was the perfect fit for the position. Plus, the interview was with a Black woman who would be my boss. This made me feel even more hopeful that I had a fighting chance.

A couple of weeks later, on New Year's Eve, I received the call saying that they wanted to offer me the internship. Not only that—they revealed to me that it was in fact a paid internship that was well above minimum wage. I was ecstatic. Emotional beyond measure, because I had been off-and-on job hunting or gig hunting as a freelancer for an entire year. To then be offered a paid internship for a job I *knew* I was going to love and be good at was the greatest blessing. It was in that moment that I knew my life was shifting and moving toward the direction of my dream. When you are finally blessed to have a breakthrough, that's when the real work starts to kick in. It is the first sign to let you know that all the tears and dedication leading up to that point have been worth it. When that happens, then it's time to prove to yourself that this is what you said you wanted. Luckily, these moments are also a reminder that the possibilities of what you want are just getting started.

When I got started at that internship, I was so grateful and eager to learn everything I possibly could, and after five months in that role, I was promoted to a full-time employee, which came with full health benefits and a major pay raise. I finally had a career, and even though it wasn't exactly video editing, my knowledge and pure love for film were enough to keep me eager to learn more about this side of the business. But most importantly, I had finally reached a financial level where I could remove myself from SSI for good. This was a moment that I recognized was bigger than my dream of being a successful video editor. I had accomplished something that many people with disabilities don't ever get the chance to. Whether it's getting off SSI or finding a dream job, these can be rare accomplishments for a person with a disability. So the fact that I was able to do both was truly a major deal. It was about my creating a life of freedom in a world that has systematically oppressed my communities. This is what the dream was really all about, it was about a *Black woman with a disability* creating a life of freedom. This was what I had been pushing myself to really achieve. This was true independence for someone like me. I was grateful beyond measure because I felt I had achieved the impossible.

Now that I was off SSI–which was a much more tedious process than I expected, but I was happy I went through it–I started to think more about the lifestyle I was wanting to achieve, rather than the career by itself. I recognized that the push to live a different life than the AOL search's prediction for me had nothing to do with a career choice. It was a life choice. I decided when I was a teenager that my life wasn't going to match that AOL search result, and I had spent all of this time using my career goals as my dream to chase. But really, it was what I felt that career could give me that the AOL search said wouldn't be possible. Sure, a career as a video editor would provide the catalyst for my new lifestyle of freedom, but what exactly would this lifestyle entail? What further freedoms would I achieve by working this job?

My whole focus shifted from my dream career to my dream lifestyle. I decided to finally put myself first and focus on how to create a better lifestyle for myself, so I would never have to go through the struggles I had just come out of–ever again. I decided to focus on my health, because keeping the mentality that it was okay to sacrifice my physical health was not serving me and I needed to rearrange my priorities.

Deciding to focus on my quality of life in general was the new driver behind the work I continued to do at my job. I worked my ass off. I was there every morning, taking the bus there an hour each way, every day, rain or shine. I would work overtime and after hours, even past 7:00 p.m., and still have to take the bus for an hour to get back home. I was learning constantly and having to survive through constant staff changes. Literally every three to four months, one or more staff were getting laid off, but I made it through every time, thankfully.

The first couple of years at that job were amazing, but the long bus rides to and from the office were starting to weigh down on me, especially when the weather got ugly. Many people believe Los Angeles is always sunny, but I'm here to tell you: absolutely not. In fall and winter, it's very cold and rainy, and the streets are constantly flooding. Now, with my goals shifting to create a better life for myself, I realized it was time to move closer to the office to lessen the amount of time on the bus and see how much difference that could make toward my well-being. Here is a moment, like I was saying earlier about the universe providing a way for you when you're focused on the right part of your dream, when the universe made it possible for me to move. Once I made the decision to move closer to the office, I noticed that all of the apartments near my office were too expensive for me to live in on my own. But I could afford to split a two-bedroom apartment if I had someone I trusted to move in with me (even though I was not seeking to do a roommate situation again).

By this time, my younger brother had graduated from high school back in Stockton, and had moved to LA and taken over the lease from our older sister's studio, just a few doors down from my studio. He was helping me with caregiver services while also working at fast-food restaurants. He was drowning in expenses to maintain his own place and was looking for a way to alleviate costs. I talked to him about being roommates in a two-bedroom. He agreed; after a couple of months of apartment hunting, we found a place we could afford together, which made it possible for me to get to work more easily. We moved in, ready to start anew and open to more possibilities.

It always feels like, whenever things are going smoothly or you get into a steady routine, like I was at this job, a random occurrence will pop up out of nowhere that'll have you back to making more crucial decisions. These moments are beautiful, because they push us to grow beyond what we can imagine at any given moment. It's the universe pushing us to our next level, to avoid those dreaded but very sneaky comfort zones that we all are guilty of easily falling back into. When we make the decision to focus on our dreams, or in my case, a dream life of freedom, it comes with a level of heightened self-awareness that we are responsible for maintaining. This new responsibility to ourselves forces us to continue to make those important decisions, so we can progress at the rate the universe wants us to. And, as you work to progress in one area of your life, other areas can be affected positively too. Every element of our lives can and should be in alignment as we work to better ourselves. In this case, my knowing that the long bus route was taking a toll on me was affecting the other areas of my life, so much so that I needed to find a solution. Although having a roommate was something I never wanted to go back to doing, being there and able to help my brother, while minimizing my bus time, was the best decision. Where my life went next would be the greatest shift I've ever experienced.

Roll It Back

You can only go so far in your dream journey if you don't have those crucial conversations with yourself. There's no avoiding being honest with the reflection in the mirror if you want to reach your goals. It's hard to do, but necessary. Because if we don't become self-aware and monitor how we are treating ourselves *first*, then how well will we treat others? If you can't take good care of yourself inside and out, what makes you think you can take care of that dream car? Or that dream house? Or that dream job? The good will only last so long until the bad shows up and rears its ugly head, smack-dab in the middle of your journey. And it will consistently show up until you do the work to do better for yourself first. Don't be scared, ashamed, prideful, embarrassed at what you see and feel in that mirror: embrace it, tackle it, whoop its ass, and fight for the better version of you, because you're worth it.

Know the difference between your ego saying, "I don't like something," and your spirit telling you, "You should not engage with that." Ego will have you believe you deserve more of something you never worked for, that you never put hours into achieving—it will have you wanting the same results as a person who did do those countless hours of work. This is you trying to treat your dream like a get-rich-quick scheme. Sorry, y'all, that's not how this grind works. Putting in the hours, days, years of work is *unavoidable*—you *must do the work* to get to the dream. I know social media creates misconstrued thinking that you can become successful fast. While for some people success does happen fast, but please believe it's a shit-show roller coaster to stay there. When you put in the work, you build up those tools that can keep you successful and push you to grow to a new level every time. There's no avoiding it, so get that ego out of the way; it's just causing traffic. Now, when your spirit says "You should not engage in that," that's because it's warning you that the thing is not good for your mental, physical, or spiritual health. These are quality-of-life decisions made to avoid long-term issues.

This isn't rooted in what you feel you deserve; it's rooted in keeping yourself safe.

You have to have self-awareness and willingness to work to decide what the dream you're chasing is really all about. It goes from "What do I want?" to "*Why* do I want this?" If we don't know the true "why" behind what we're chasing, we will constantly feel like we're doing work yet going nowhere. Being honest with yourself during the process of recognizing your why is crucial so it can help focus your goals in the right direction. So, as you continue to reflect on your journey, stop and ask yourself, "*Why* do I want this? *Why* do I want to achieve this in this way? *Why* does this keep calling me to accomplish it?"

Get Rolling

Tough Talk Ain't Easy

But we have to do it—especially during the times when we feel like we can't catch a break. That usually means we have to self-evaluate and tell ourselves the *real*, and not just the stuff we want to hear.

Here are some ways to recognize when it's time for tough talk.

1. **If you are having more days of struggle than relief.** Yes, everyone goes through tough times, but when those struggles are outweighing the moments of joy, it's time to reevaluate what's going on in the moment. Write a list, if you must, to recognize what those struggles are so you can have a starting place for what needs to be taken care of.

2. **When your basic life necessities aren't being managed properly.** When our basic needs aren't met or managed properly, it does nothing but continue to cause stress and make matters worse. It's time to think hard about what caused the mess and why it's not getting any better. I'd say, start by making a list and ask people in your foundation if there's something you're overlooking. Many times, with trauma, we suppress the experiences to avoid facing the pain, but that's where your foundation can come in and be there to help you discover your challenges, even if you aren't ready to face them.

3. **When everything you're trying simply isn't working.** No matter how hard you're trying, or no matter what solutions you're coming up with, if it isn't working, it's time to *stop*. Sit still and think deeply about what your motivation is. Recognize that you may need help from outside of yourself. We can't do it all by ourselves. We need help. Even if it's not a literal other person, but instead podcasts, books, music, community programs, or local services, get creative and think outside the box. Anything helpful that isn't your own brain or ego can do wonders.

The New Responsibility

When you become aware of the real motivations behind your dreams, it creates an internal energy shift that causes you to elevate everything you've been working on.

Here are some ways to honor the new responsibility.

1. **What areas of your life do you feel could use some help or attention?** Whether it's implementing regular self-care routines, setting up payment plans to manage debt, learning better time management skills, signing up for therapy, etc., you must give those areas attention and create a solution to better handle stresses. You don't have to tackle them all together and all at once. Just choose one and work from there.

2. **Do you feel any positive progress is happening?** If so, wonderful! That means your energy is shifting in the right direction. If not, stop again and reevaluate. Are you trying to solve too much too fast? Is your focus on everything else and not yourself and your needs? Really think about those things, refer back to the list you made in the previous section, and get back focused on what you're needing to accomplish.

3. **If everything is going great, what do you do next?** You simply maintain the systems you put in place to get you to this point, while continuing to learn more ways to better your life and implement more things that keep you in a positive space. That way, when it's time to make another decision, it doesn't feel as disruptive as it has before.

Chapter 7

IT'S SITTING PRETTY, BABY

"I guess I can start a YouTube channel. People have always wanted to know how I live positively with a disability. Maybe I can make videos on that."

I had been working at my job for almost two years by this time. It had been an amazing learning experience so far. I was learning something new every day about the distribution side of the film industry, which isn't often taught in school. I tended to keep to myself because I was so focused on wanting to do my job well. Plus, there were rumors of the company finding out about an employee's social media posts and them getting in trouble for it. That told me to stick to myself, do my job, and go home. Whenever there was a meeting, I avidly took notes on terms that were repeatedly used, projects that were being reviewed for the company, and shows or movies everyone was talking about in casual conversation. I would go back to my desk, and for anything I wasn't familiar with, I would Google the terms and memorize their meanings so I could better understand what was happening in the meeting, and ultimately learn to do my job better. Then I would go home and watch the shows or movies that were recently talked about, so I could be aware of what was happening in the office conversations. Because I was new to everything in corporate culture and in the distribution industry itself, I knew I had to do my best at keeping up and applying effort, because I couldn't risk losing this job.

Whenever you get an opportunity that you feel you may not have been prepared for, just know there might be some extra work you have to do to keep up, and that's okay. It's not a sign that you're not deserving, because, if the company felt like you weren't qualified, they wouldn't have hired you. You deserve to be there. Now, all you must do is work to stay there. So, if it means you have to do extra research while in the office, ask coworkers some questions, or do work that applies to your job outside of the office and working extra hours, you may have to do that. The benefit of working a corporate job is that there is usually room to grow within the company. This means there are continuous opportunities to gain more knowledge, power, and of course money, so long as you're showing improvement and progress. However, there will be times or predicaments in which your work may not be enough to some supervisors, and that's when juggling the "politics" of a corporate environment comes into play. Or it could be just the push you need to elevate to the next phase in your life.

By this time, I was on my second supervisor. Remember, they were laying people off left and right in this company, and although I was glad I was making it through every cut, I was affected by it because I had to adjust to new coworkers and, this time, to a new boss. Although this new boss was a nice lady, she wasn't the boss who'd hired me when I applied as an intern and who I'd built a relationship with, so it was a challenge to get used to this new person. Her supervising style was very different from my previous boss's—she had been much more relaxed and had trust in my skillset and abilities to do quality work and meet deadlines, whereas the new boss was a lot more impatient with my working style, and needed reports for everything I was doing on a much more frequent basis than I was used to. Also, she was in cahoots with a coworker of mine who had been a bit standoffish toward me because she felt I wasn't doing enough to figure out the details of my job. This is where knowing your working and learning style matters. Although I felt like I was doing my part, I was still more of an "ask questions, visual learner" type of person. I was instructed by my previous boss to ask this particular coworker for answers about anything that I couldn't find on the internet—basically more in-office-specific systems and programming, all of which I knew nothing about and had no formal training on. So I asked questions or needed to be shown a lot of things, which until this fateful meeting, I had no idea was getting on that girl's nerves.

I was casually sitting at my desk one day, doing my work, when my new boss called me into her office. When I went inside, she shut the door. I knew this was about to be a serious conversation. I was very confused because I had no idea what it could be about. She proceeded to tell me how appreciative she was for having me as part of the team and that I was a valuable person to the company, but I wasn't producing the quality of work she wanted and in the format she wanted to see things in. On top of that, the coworker she was in cahoots with had been complaining to her directly about my work, with no mention to me that I was doing anything subpar to begin with. She then showed me how to "properly" format my work on her computer using Microsoft Excel (which, by the way, might be one of the most challenging office programs ever). Anywho, she ended the meeting with the tone and energy of, "If you don't get this right moving forward, we may have to let you go." I left her office livid. I couldn't express my emotion on the job, so I had to hold it in for the rest of the day, until I could call my mom after work. I was in tears. I was upset by this for so many reasons. I was hurt because, until I had to work with this new boss, my quality or ability to do my work was never in question. I felt that, as long as I had been doing the work and meeting any deadlines and no one, to my knowledge, had been complaining about my work performance, then what really was the problem? Then to find out that there was someone complaining about me behind my back, saying that I could do better, felt shady, especially since she was going directly to my boss without even giving me a chance to fix the issue first. But what was even more upsetting was that, if that lady was ready to fire me, she was able to take *everything* I had worked so hard for with just the snap of her fingers or ego. She had control of my entire livelihood because she was my boss. Not because I was a bad employee—only because, if she felt like firing me, she could, without any regard for my future.

Had she fired me that day, I would have had to go back on SSI and to freelancing to try to make ends meet, on top of now being responsible for keeping a roof over my and my brother's head. To know I had to go back to job hunting, and maybe not even have the rare opportunity to find another job at this level as a person with a disability, would've felt like an impossible task. It had taken me a year to even find the internship, which then took another five months before it turned into the position I was in. I didn't have that type of time to spare anymore. I had to figure out a plan and figure it out fast, because my new boss and this coworker, I felt, had it out for me. And if I made one more mistake in their eyes, it was over for me at this job. With my mom and I both having hustler mentalities, my mom asked me, "What could you do to make your own money outside of your job? That way, you're not solely dependent on this job to maintain your livelihood."

I thought for a second.

"Well, all I know how to do is produce and edit videos. But to find music artists, then pitch them ideas, isn't guaranteed work that I'll always be able to find."

We both went silent.

"Can you sell something? Make something to sell? Or maybe produce videos that don't require music?"

I thought some more.

"I guess I can start a YouTube channel. People have always wanted to know how I live positively with a disability. Maybe I can make videos on that."

"Can you make money off YouTube?"

"Oh yeah! People are becoming millionaires off there."

"Then it sounds like you need to start a YouTube channel."

And that's how *Sitting Pretty* was born. For the next couple of weeks, every day after work, I would go online and work on my channel: filling out all the information needed to set up my account, watching other people's videos with tips on how to start a channel and applying that to my setup, writing out video topic ideas, and finding tools I had around my own place that I could use to start filming my videos with. I started my channel by recording on the weekends, because that was the only way I could catch the natural light that came through my window and use it as my "lighting setup." The windowsill was my "camera tripod." My "backdrop" was my bare living room with the kitchen next to it, in which I always had to coordinate with my brother to not leave his room so I could record. My "camera" was an iPad mini, my "microphone" was the one built into the iPad, and my "editing software" was iMovie. As a trained video editor, iMovie was the worst possible option to edit videos, but I had to use something. I used what I had and made the best of it until I could save the money and grow from there. We have to be sure that we don't let perfectionism steal our dreams. I always tell people who want to launch anything, especially a YouTube channel, that the videos don't have to be perfect right away. You don't need to break the bank or wait months to save money to buy the best camera, audio equipment, backdrop setup, or editing program—all you need is to use whatever you already have, or whatever you can afford, and then grow from there. And, because it will be your first video, no matter how fancy it is at launch, it's more than likely still only going to get a bare minimum number of views anyway. We can't compare our starting-off points to someone else's five-year run at creating content. Take the pressure off yourself and simply start making content. Your motivation and dreams depend on it.

Every day, I had gone back to work after that meeting with my new boss feeling more motivated than ever. Not to do my work at the office, but to create content outside of the office, to prove no one would have the power to control my livelihood. A couple of weeks went by, and my channel was almost ready to launch. I was still brainstorming ideas for videos while at work when, one day, I caught my new boss in the hallway. I was approaching her to ask a question when I noticed she was crying. She told me that the company had just fired her. An array of thoughts flooded my mind. I returned to my desk to give her a moment alone. Shortly after that, the coworker who had complained about my work behind my back came to my desk to let me know she was quitting the company and going to a new job, and today was her last day at the office. And just like that, in one day, in a matter of minutes, both people who had given me trouble at my job, and had inadvertently threatened my future at the company, were both leaving the company for good.

When I got home that night, I called my mom. I told her what had happened at the office, and she was equally as shocked as I was. And then she said, "God is always in control." I knew at that moment that I had to launch this channel. This was exactly what I was supposed to be doing next on my journey toward my new dream lifestyle for myself. This was the window of opportunity, where I knew I had to build this channel to take back my power over my livelihood, because whoever my next boss was would never get the opportunity to feel like they had control over my future. When I look back at this time, it was such an obvious God wink from the universe. They were making space and assuring me that everything was going to be okay. I had so many thoughts and emotions. I felt bad for my boss because losing your job is a terrifying experience, plus she had just moved to LA while all of her family and friends stayed on the East Coast. Yet at the same time I felt relieved that both were leaving while I got to stay. This gave me reassurance that my income, my foundation, wasn't going anywhere, and my life was no longer on the brink of falling off completely. I still had time to provide for myself, and now take ownership over my life in a way I hadn't realized I needed to in order to secure my future. I still felt a bit nervous because I didn't know how much more time I had at the job, since the layoffs were clearly still happening. I had to take advantage of juggling a job and a channel as much as I could. Plus, with having to relearn how to work with another new boss, I didn't know what to expect. I then felt an overwhelming sense of motivation to get the YouTube channel launched officially. I knew that, as soon as I launched, I wouldn't be working a traditional job ever again if I could help it.

I launched my channel. My first video was a recap on my first trip to Miami with my cousins. It was a great video. It definitely had room to improve, but I loved it. After the first video, I dedicated myself to posting at least one video a week, and to do my best to post on a consistent day of the week and at a consistent time. Between working full-time, taking care of personal needs, and my social life (which I make a priority for my sanity), I knew that was all I had the bandwidth to produce at the time.

After posting my first few videos, I went through a stage of needing to find my voice in my channel. How did I want to showcase my disability lifestyle? How could I keep it authentic to me? What was the message I wanted to give that I felt I hadn't seen shared by other creators with disabilities? Doing the deep dive behind the intention of creating my content is what really shaped my identity as a creator. I knew I had to be true to my voice and feelings. If that meant I was drunk at a party, I'd show it. If I was cursing every other word, then keep it. If I were expressing myself and was crying, I'd leave it in the edit. For me, it was most important to always be as authentic as possible to my experience and expression. Even my mom asked, "Are you sure you should be cussing in your videos? What if brands don't want to work with you because of it?"

And I told her, "Then those brands aren't right for me. I don't want to be rewarded for being someone I'm not. Brands will know by watching my content who they are asking to work with. No surprises." That was important to me. What also was important were the moments or stories I chose *not* to share on my channel. I wanted to maintain a certain level of privacy for myself. There are experiences and people in life that aren't the business of anyone else. The internet will only know what I share with them. I protect myself by managing what I'm willing to share, and whatever I do choose to share, it will always be authentic to me. Once I really got in the groove of consistently posting videos unique to my experience as a person with a disability, I started to grow an audience online. It was amazing to witness people leaving me comments, the faithful people watching and liking every video, the private messages about how my content was helping them, and every month, the number of subscribers and views would get larger and larger. This is when I knew that I was doing something bigger for people than just entertaining them with my wild nights and colorful stories. I was really affecting people's lives. This was bigger than me now. This was my life's purpose. *This* is what God wanted me to do all this time. This was to be the catalyst to creating the lifestyle of freedom I'd been chasing after all this time.

I recognized that my purpose was "To showcase disability lifestyle in a fun, fly, sexy kind of way in every piece of content I create or project I'm part of. To represent disability authentically in all areas of my life, to encourage fellow people with disabilities that the life they desire is possible and to dismantle the ableist perspective that has been put on our community."

And I've been doing that now for almost a decade. My channel was able to launch me into a multitude of opportunities I know I never would've had the chance to experience by sitting behind my desk at my job, trying to please a boss I wasn't getting along with. Many of these opportunities were things I never thought I could do, but I always went into them open to trying, because the purpose of my work was bigger than my own lack of knowledge about the process. Since I launched my channel, I've become a public speaker, model, product ambassador, author, serial entrepreneur, disability advocate, forever a content creator, and the most unexpected career path of all: an actress. I had no idea where any of these paths were really going to take my life, but no matter what it was, so long as it wasn't going to compromise my moral compass, I was open to figuring out how to best execute in the opportunity. But I never could have imagined how taking that leap of faith to try acting for the first time would take my life in a direction I never saw coming.

Roll It Back

Launching a new career path all on your own is a very intimidating and, for many people, a very scary process. I felt motivated to work to prevent others from taking my livelihood away from me—prevent them from bringing me back to a lifestyle I had worked hard not to have again. This made the process feel necessary to my well-being regardless of the amount of work it was or how much fear I might've had. But I know that's not everyone else's process.

The most common thing I recognized from people I'd share my journey with was that they had the desire to follow a similar path as I had, yet they were scared because they knew that whatever brand they were working to launch couldn't be perfect right away. Perfect doesn't exist. Perfectionism is a procrastination tool we use because the deeper reason for wanting everything to be just right before executing is fear. Fear of rejection, or fear of failure, or fear of others' opinion, and, truthfully, all those feelings hold us back from going after our dreams. Letting go of the idea that your brand or vision needs to be materialized perfectly will do wonders in your life. I'm not saying you should settle for a lower level of quality for your work; however, if whatever you're working on can be completed using materials around your home or making the necessary investments in creating products you might want to sell, then launch it. The benefit of not waiting to be perfect is that it allows you the opportunity to grow and build an audience that will support you through your growth. And as you grow, you can continue to tap in with your audience, who can help guide you on where to go next with your brand.

Keep in mind that you ultimately always have control of your brand. You can take suggestions from others, but really, you can do and share as much as you feel like sharing. Do not feel pressured by social media or your audience to give or produce something you don't want to. You should always have control over your brand because you have to be happy with what you produce at all times. Be mindful not to fall into what you assume makes brands successful, and focus solely on the principles you live by for your brand. We don't know the intricacies of other peoples' lives or journeys, so to compare what you're doing with what others are doing is a slippery slope. Everyone starts their dreams with just a vision in their heads, then they put in time and hard work, and grow every day—that's the process and there's no escaping it, so don't feel intimidated by other people's work; focus on what you bring to the world. There is an audience for everyone. You don't need to capture every single person's attention, just the attention of those who understand your vision best.

Get Rolling

Work It

The wild thing about living a life dedicated to making decisions to create a dream lifestyle for yourself is that you will often come across opportunities and, even if you're not entirely prepared for it, they will be too good to pass up.

When those moments happen, here are some tips to get you feeling more comfortable in the opportunity:

1. **It's never too late to prepare.** Once you're given a new opportunity that you feel unprepared for, start preparing immediately. Whether it's note-taking and Google searching or taking a class in your free time or finding a mentor in the space, do whatever you need to

do. You'll start to gain the knowledge you need on top of the experience, and this will help you manage the new opportunity much more efficiently.

2. **You are worthy.** If ever given a new opportunity you feel unprepared for, do your best to affirm to yourself that you are worthy. It can be tough to accept good things in our lives if we feel inadequate, but we have to focus on the reality that the opportunity was given to us regardless. Stay encouraged to know that you are deserving of any opportunity you want that comes your way.

3. **Enjoy the process.** When experiencing an opportunity, the best thing we can do is fully immerse ourselves in the process. Enjoy everything you are learning, enjoy the extra work to prepare, enjoy the people involved, etc. Embrace everything the new opportunity is giving to you, and before you know it, you will be a professional in your new space.

Work With What You've Got

Social media is one of the greatest beasts to tackle and manage in our lives. It's hard because the whole platform is an illusion of successes and perfectionism in ways that can be completely toxic and unrealistic. Don't let social media or perfectionism stop you from pursuing your goals. Here are some tips on how to recognize you're worrying too much about external expectations:

1. **Are you stalling because of others' opinions?** I do
    believe in receiving healthy, constructive feedback
    from people whose opinions we trust, *but* if we are
    concerned about the opinions of people we don't know
    or people who don't love us, and we are fighting for
    their approval, we need to reflect on our motivation
    behind why we're not pursuing our own desires instead.

2. **Are you waiting for perfect?** Rude awakening: there is
    no such thing as perfect. Perfectionism is an excuse we
    use to stall our pursuits because deep down we aren't
    ready for the unforeseen possibilities. *But*, if there's
    anything you want to pursue, accept that it will never be
    "perfect" enough before it's time to launch the pursuit.
    As Nike would say, "Just Do It."

3. **Are you ready for success?** Whenever we talk about the
    fear that comes with pursuing dreams, we often focus
    on everything that can go wrong in the process, *but* very
    rarely do we discuss the fear associated when we think
    about the possibility of everything going right. And I
    believe more people are scared of what can go right
    than are scared of what can go wrong. We do have to
    think about what can go right and not be intimidated
    by the possibility. Because, when it goes right, it's an
    opportunity for growth and change in the best way.
    Don't be afraid of it—embrace it, because it's what your
    heart desires.

Chapter 8

AUNTIE'S IN A MOVIE

"What it would mean to represent people with disabilities, and particularly Black people with disabilities, in a leading role was more important than my own fear."

My job was finally at a place I liked. My new boss was the best! Such a drastic difference from the lady before her, and I was very happy. My new boss and I had really built such a strong bond during this time that, to this day, I still consider her a great personal mentor of mine. And I was able to continue to grow my channel while simultaneously working my full-time job. I created a real schedule for myself to be able to balance work and build my YouTube channel and social media presence. My full-time job would serve as the monetary asset to fund my basic needs—rent, food, utilities. It also paid for recording equipment, like camera, audio, and lighting, and any experience expenses needed to create content, like parties, makeup, clothes, events, etc. My YouTube channel would be the asset that would grow so that, eventually, I would not need the full-time job anymore. Any income I made from YouTube or social media, which at the beginning was very little, I would feed back into the production of my channel.

The benefit of my channel was that it allowed other types of paid opportunities to open up for me that I didn't intend to pursue. But once the opportunities came up, I took advantage, because it was about the purpose of disability representation

in all facets of the entertainment and beauty industries. For instance, I was always able to do my public speaking events (something very new for me) on the weekends, or use vacation and sick days saved up at the office for any opportunities pertaining to my YouTube during a work week—sometimes not the most admirable thing to do, but it was the only way for me to do both, and I needed to do both.

Everything was finally going as planned. It was a lot of work juggling both careers, but it was what I needed to do in order to build the lifestyle of my dreams. That's where I feel hustle culture does get it right. We assume that working a traditional job while pursuing a dream is counterintuitive. Where the saying goes, "Don't have a plan B, because it's a distraction from plan A." In many ways this is true, but plan A can still be your focus even while you're working somewhere that isn't fully aligned with that plan—and to do so in order to maintain your basic living necessities. There is nothing wrong with doing both.

As a result of my consistency in my YouTube channel *Sitting Pretty*, my audience was growing at a consistent pace. I was learning, during this time, that I didn't have to force myself or push myself to do anything extra in my career to have success. New types of career opportunities all came to me organically. Once you're in the flow of your purpose and focused on your dreams, what is meant for you will come your way without you even needing to seek it. That is something to really believe and hold onto if you are in pursuit of dreams. I'm a firm believer in exercising other opportunities that come your way, because sometimes those opportunities can open up a creativity that'll be useful to your plan A. Or your plan A can morph into something more expansive, or something else altogether, because a new opportunity sparked your interest or creativity more. However, that's why it's crucial, regardless of the type of opportunity, to still be steadfast in your "why." It is very easy to fall into the trap of trying a new opportunity because it's "fancier" or makes you more money quicker than what you're working on currently, but if it's completely the opposite of your heart-driven "why," those opportunities will never last, and more than likely will leave you feeling completely off-track with yourself. I was focused only on doing the work to push for disability representation and inclusion in the beauty and entertainment industries via my content on *Sitting Pretty*. And, as a result, more opportunities that would lead me further into my purpose came my way. Although I had an agent, she was only focused on getting me film, TV, and commercial opportunities. Anything extra, like brand content collaborations, public speaking, or modeling, would come to me directly.

Until, one day, my agent finally called and told me that a pair of independent filmmakers were working on a project and specifically looking for a young Black woman who was a wheelchair user to be the lead actress in their film. It was titled *Give Me Liberty*. I had never acted a day in my life before this moment. Sure, I'd played myself as an influencer in comedy sketches, but real dialogue, real character development, real movie stuff, not at all. This was the first opportunity I received where I actually felt intimidated. Because I had so much experience in TV production, the art of acting was a career I always had extreme reverence for, but never wanted to attempt without giving it its due diligence and taking it seriously. But the opportunity was presented, and I figured it would do more damage to myself or create regret if I didn't at least try. Since the opportunity was there, I auditioned, with the motive and understanding that if I were to book this role, what it would mean to represent people with disabilities, and particularly Black people with disabilities, in a leading role was more important than my own fear.

I submitted my audition video. I had no hope or expectation of booking it. I just sent it knowing I at least tried my best. A week later, I found out I had booked the role. Imagine my shock. But luckily, in true independent filmmaking fashion, the filmmakers were not in a position to go into production anytime soon. Two years of preproduction later, after multiple instances of stop-and-go regarding when they needed me to arrive at the film shoot, and countless Skype calls with the filmmakers to develop my character, it was time to start working toward getting to Milwaukee to shoot. When it was time to go, I learned I had to be in Milwaukee for over three straight weeks. This then presented another challenge: how I was going to explain all of this to my boss. And not only the opportunity to be in a film, but also explain to her that the opportunity came as a result of building a whole separate career outside of the office, doing influencer work advocating for people with disabilities. I had finally gotten to a place where I enjoyed my job, and in large part because of her. And being gone over three weeks while being able to keep my job looked more impossible by the minute. Plus, I was at the point in the filmmaking process where backing out of the film was *not* an option. I had to accept the scary possibility that I would have to quit my job and come up with a plan for my income when I got back. My only hope was banking on the relationship that I'd built with my new boss—that she would understand and help support me in finding a solution for me to come back to my job after I was done filming.

Breaking the news to my boss about everything I had been working on outside of the office, while also asking for support and understanding, was one of the scariest decisions of my life. I had to tell her. You can imagine the shocked look on her face when I finally spilled the beans to her, in an effort to drop the final bomb that I was requesting time off from work that I knew I hadn't saved up. But, after a few conversations and some divine help, my time off was approved (they reduced my hours to part-time for the duration of filming), and I was off to Milwaukee to act for the very first time.

This was one of the most divine moments of my life, where I felt I literally watched the universe move mountains for me to help me pursue the next phase of my career while also keeping my basic needs protected. While at times things may look impossible, you would be pleasantly surprised at how *possible* your dreams really are. This is how I've learned that we cannot let fear get in the way of our progress. Fear is a very strong feeling, but it's only a feeling. It's not real. Sure, there are some instinctual fears that we should listen to, if we are at the edge of a steep cliff without a parachute or safety net– yes, turn back around and go in a different direction that is safe. But if the decision we have to make is not life-or-death, and we recognize that fear is keeping us hesitant about making a decision, we should consider building the courage to move past the fear.

Part of moving past that fear is considering the factors that are working in your favor to help you take those leaps. For me, it was the great relationship with my new boss and the side hustle of a social media presence that I built for myself that helped. Sometimes all you need are one or two things to work in your favor to ultimately give you courage. Yes, it is very scary in the moment, but know that feeling of fear will subside and make you even more courageous the next time you're fearful of making a decision. You just need to prove it to yourself once that you can survive it—trust me, it's worth taking the chance.

Filming *Give Me Liberty* in Milwaukee was one of the most unique and life-changing experiences I have ever had. Because this was an independent film, it took a lot of "glue bottles and Popsicle sticks" to keep this film together. But the beauty of it was witnessing the entire cast and crew being willing to wear multiple hats, to work as much as we needed to no matter how long it took, all for the sake of completing this film we all believed in. When you are working on a set like this one, the best thing you can do is be the best at your part of the process. And that's how I went into every shoot day. I knew I had no real acting experience, but this entire cast and crew were depending on me to give the best performance for each take, to make all this extreme work everyone was putting themselves through worth it. Although the filmmakers never made me feel pressured to perform at extreme heights, that was the responsibility I felt obligated to take on. Every day I would go on set and say a prayer to myself: "Lauren, give all that you have to give. Do the best that you can. As long as you know you did the best that you could, then that's a job well done." I didn't have any techniques or skillsets to lean into to help me act, just my pure instinct and what I'd learned from studying actors as a fan of film and TV my whole life.

Since I was blessed to still be employed at my job, I also had to find ways to manage the obligations for my coworkers back in LA. Whenever I wasn't on set, whether it meant waking up early, going to bed late, or spending an entire off day working on my job back in LA, that's what I did. I would take meetings during my breaks while filming, answer emails on my phone or in the hotel after I wrapped on set. I still had my obligations to the office and, just like I would tell myself before every scene to do my best, I applied it to my job in LA too. When you're on a mission for the dream life you desire. there will be moments when your decisions will take a lot out of you to keep going. But when you keep your "why," your motivation behind the work, at the forefront, you will start to find the time you need to put the work toward the dream. You'll start thinking outside the box and dedicate the time you have, no matter how much or how little, toward whatever you need to accomplish that day—because doing absolutely nothing is no longer an option.

After filming, I went right back to work in the office. I was proud of what I had accomplished and could only hope that *Give Me Liberty* would finish being made, and if so, that I had at least done a good job. I was so nervous that the filmmakers would go into the editing room and feel like they'd made a mistake by taking a chance on a non-actor. A few months went by, and I was asked to come back to Milwaukee for reshoots. Luckily, this time, it was only for a couple of days, and I just used my paid time off at the job to go back. While I was there, the filmmakers were raving about how well I had done in my scenes. A complete shock and relief, with a little skepticism, flooded my brain when hearing this. I wasn't sure how to take it all in, because I still hadn't seen anything I had filmed, so I had to trust that they weren't just being nice. Then they shared a secret with me. The filmmakers whispered to me, "Lolo, we can't make this public yet, but we got accepted into Sundance." That's when I knew we had done something great, and that I had made the right decision to gamble on myself and be in the film. Sundance Film Festival is one of the most prestigious and largest film festivals dedicated to independent films in the United States. Some of the most loved, award-winning, and A-list celebrities got their big break at Sundance. It can be career- and life-changing all in the same breath if your film is a hit at the festival. *Give Me Liberty* was headed to Sundance. This was the moment I knew every decision leading up to this point was about to be worth it, my

life was about to change. A couple of months later, we went to
Sundance. Every screening was sold out, packed with viewers
and press, and the Q & A's we hosted after every screening
were a success. Top press outlets like the *Hollywood Reporter*
and *RogerEbert.com* praised our film and, thankfully, our
acting too. It was at Sundance that I recognized I was officially
an actor, and a great actor at that. People would stop me
and my castmates as we roamed the festival grounds, giving
us compliments on our performances and asking to take
pictures. Little did we know, this was just the beginning of a
ride that would change all our lives.

A few months later, we got the call that we'd also been
accepted into a director's category at the Cannes Film
Festival, one of the most prestigious film festivals in the world,
and we were all invited to attend. The festival is located in
Cannes in the South of France, and it was one of the most
beautiful cities I had ever seen. It was my first time flying
internationally, and it was worth every minute of the ten-hour
flight to Paris, the one-hour flight to Nice, and the forty-five-
minute car ride to our hotel in Cannes. We had a blast! Shortly
after our time in Cannes, it was time for the United States
theatrical release of the film. Because of the indie budget, we
were limited to certain cities, but the impact was still great
enough to affect the masses in the way the film was intended
to. We were constantly in the press, with reviews from *The
New York Times*, the *LA Times*, and *The Wrap* Magazine, and,
to this day, *Give Me Liberty* holds an 89 percent rating on
Rotten Tomatoes. Audiences were loving it.

After some months of festivals, theater premieres, and
press junkets, we received the greatest news yet. *Give Me
Liberty* had been nominated for four Film Independent Spirit
Awards. The Film Independent Spirit Awards are the most
sought-after awards dedicated to independent films. Of

the four nominations *Give Me Liberty* received, one was a nomination for my performance in the Best Supporting Actress category, alongside fellow nominees Jennifer Lopez and Octavia Spencer. And I had done all of this work promoting the film in all of these places while still working at my job in LA. From Sundance in January 2019 to the Spirit Awards in February 2020, I was juggling my now-budding acting career and my LA job, working remotely while traveling. During that time, I would go from chauffeured car service and paid hotel stays and flights one week, to hours-long bus rides, paying rent, and eight-hour-plus workdays in LA the next. How I was able to do it still amazes me, and doing it all while taking care of myself and my disability was truly the universe looking out for me. It was the most exciting time in my life. To have my career changing in front of me, and balancing my "old" life with this new one, left me at my next crossroads and my greatest decision—ever.

Roll It Back

What's happened in my career makes this time in life one of the wildest ever. Because, when you finally allow yourself to go for a dream and live in complete faith, the universe opens up to you in an expansive way, in a way you never could've dreamed of. And the only way to get to the next stage of your journey is by sticking to your "why" the entire time. That's why it's important to be diligent in knowing what your "why" is, to inform you of what your next move will be—even when the next move doesn't make any rational sense to whatever you thought your plan was. Your "why" allows you to feel more secure in your decisions moving forward while having faith that you're going in the right direction. When you fully focus on your "why," you'll learn just how possible your dreams really are.

This time in my life showed me the importance of divine timing. That no matter how much the odds are seemingly against you, whatever is meant for you will be for you to have. Opportunities will show up in ways you never expected, and that's why we always have to keep trying. Be open to other ways to get to your desired goals. There is no one way to do anything; we must be open to always trying. Sometimes, our plans to achieve our dreams are limited by our fear of getting something wrong or wasting our time. So we rely on one way to do something, thinking that it will give us a more guaranteed, less risky, and more failure-proof chance at going after what we want. Sorry to share this with you, but even the safe route doesn't make the journey easier. If anything, it makes the journey longer and more boring. Having to make life-changing decisions is scary, yet it's necessary, because deep down, you know it's worth it.

Get Rolling

Be Open

Decision-making is a skill that should be constantly applied to everything you do to create the results you desire. Part of exercising the skill of decision-making is learning how to make decisions around opportunities that are completely brand new to you. That means decisions that give you that feeling of "This just feels like something I want to try," even if you have no solid information or experience in the field of the opportunity.

My suggestion is to be open to the opportunities because you never know where they may lead you:

1. **There's more than one way to do anything.** In hustle
   culture, we tend to believe that there is only one way
   to achieve our goals, when in reality that's not true.
   There are multiple ways to make a tuna sandwich, drive
   a long distance, or work a job—why would the paths
   to our dreams be any different? If a new opportunity
   comes your way, take a moment to evaluate what the
   opportunity is. For me, as long as it doesn't compromise
   your moral compass, isn't illegal, doesn't harm innocent
   people, and is in alignment with your "why," then I
   suggest trying it. Had I been stubborn and believed that
   I was only a YouTuber and YouTube was the only way I
   wanted to achieve success, I would never have gotten
   the opportunities to have the experiences I had.

2. **Exercise new gifts.** We all have talents within us that we
   either believe we are not good enough to pursue, or
   simply haven't considered at all, for whatever reason.
   I suggest you tap into those gifts anyway and see
   what can come of them by at least trying them. I don't
   believe we have gifts inside of us that we aren't meant
   to share with others or experience during our lifetimes.
   They don't all have to be pursued as career paths,
   but some other gifts may help you become greater at
   your ultimate purpose. Acting was a gift that I allowed
   myself to finally explore, even in the midst of feeling
   inadequate because of my own self-inflicted sense of
   limitation about my talents. But once I moved past that,
   I learned that I was a really talented actor—a gift that
   would've forever been ignored had I not given it a try.

3. **Find your rhythm.** When you're juggling multiple
   careers—the dream career and the career you need to

make a living–things can become overwhelming very fast. The best way to balance it all is to be open to new ways to conquer tasks. Everything has to get done, but remember, it doesn't all have to be done in a day. My suggestion is to dedicate at least one to two hours of work toward your dream career every day. You'll have to get creative and, in some cases, sacrifice to find that time, but that's what makes it fun. Listen to podcasts that teach you new skills involving your dream career on your way to the office instead of listening to music; sign up for the weekend workshop you've been needing to take while you're waiting in the Chipotle line for lunch; or put the kids to bed early after work so you can have the remainder of the evening to work on your dream.

Be Brave

Being fearful is no joke. Fear is a tricky feeling because, in many ways, we never know if the fear is truly protecting us from harm, or if it's just an excuse to not try. That's the toughest part to decipher when experiencing fear in the midst of decision-making.

Here are my tips to help work through your fears when you need to make big life decisions:

1. **Is it life or death?** And I mean that literally. Will making this decision actually be a matter of life or death? Similar to the cliff example earlier in the chapter, if it's not a similar circumstance, then more than likely whatever decision you have to make, you'll survive at the end, so do what you really feel is best for you. If taking the leap does risk your survival, whether that means losing your

home, your medical care, or anything else extreme, then it's time to get creative on how to make it all work.

2. **Know what's best.** When battling with your fear during the time of deciding, you have to be absolutely clear about what "best for you" really means to your life. For instance, if you're strapped for cash and an opportunity comes that can help pay some important bills, but you know that, if you went through with the opportunity, you would live with extreme regret because it compromises your morals—then choosing to still take the opportunity isn't doing what's best. Because yes, the money will temporarily solve some bills, but the regret will be much harder to solve and will negatively affect your decision-making moving forward. Trust this: the Universe or God would never need you to compromise yourself to survive; they will always come through, even if you don't see it right away.

3. **Accept not knowing.** Fear happens in decision-making because, when we are faced with an opportunity we want to take advantage of, in many cases we may not have all the details we need to make us feel comfortable about making the decision. Welp, get used to it. The power of decision-making isn't always going to be comfortable, especially for life-changing-level decisions. All we can do is evaluate the information we do have, do more research if possible, and focus on how making the decision makes you feel. Sometimes on paper everything will look perfect and great, but if something about it still doesn't make you joyous—pay attention to that. And other times, we may have limited information and yet, it makes us feel happy and alive—pay attention to that also. Whichever feeling aligns with your "best for you," lean toward that choice.

Chapter 9
THIS SH*T IS WILD

"...but who is looking out for you?"

Was I going to quit my job and pursue acting and content creation work full time? I had to weigh my options. By this time, my brother and I had moved out of our shared apartment and I had gotten my own place, so I was back to having all responsibilities on me. Although I was receiving praise and accolades as an actor, I wasn't getting paid anything extra beyond my initial fee to play the role. Although it was exciting and fun in the moment, I had to be real. I wasn't making enough money as an actor yet to cover my living expenses. But acting and content creator work was taking me in the direction I wanted to go to have my dream lifestyle. It was in line with my purpose of disability representation, and it came naturally to me. It ultimately made me happy to do the work. I was booking more speaking gigs and auditioning regularly now, but I hadn't made money off anything yet. I had more opportunities in limbo than I had guaranteed work. My office job was guaranteed income. None of my basic needs would have to be risked, my coworkers were great, and I actually really liked the work as well. But I didn't see much growth happening for me, beyond the current position I was at within the company. Splitting my time to work a job and build this outside career was limiting my productivity in both areas. I had to trust and put my 100 percent into one or the other, otherwise I was going to physically burn out, and that was not an option.

After much prayer and a cosign from my mom, I decided
to quit my office job. I figured that, since I had some gigs lined
up already and auditions out, all I had to do was book more
speaking gigs, social media brand deals, modeling work,
and all the other social stuff to be able to make ends meet.
What I was getting paid in a one-weekend trip modeling was
more than what I made in one month working full-time at the
office. And since I'd be quitting my job, I could dedicate 100
percent of my time and energy to creating content. With my
time dedicated only to content creation, I knew my audience
would continue to grow, and booking work would be more
fruitful. I knew I was taking a major risk, but this wasn't my
first time doing so, which let me know that, whatever was to
happen next, I could handle it. My last day at the office was
March 9, 2020. Ten days later, the governor of California
issued a stay-at-home quarantine mandate as a result of the
COVID-19 pandemic.

Over the next few days, almost every other state in the
country completely shut down because of the pandemic.
That meant that every speaking gig I had lined up to cover my
expenses for the following month was canceled. I had never
seen anything like this. I checked my email and everything I
had in motion—contract executed or not—was canceled. And
I had *just quit my job!* Not only did I not have a job, but the
budding acting and content creation career went into an
immediate halt, because those careers involved being around
large groups of people, which was no longer a possibility. As
we all remember, nothing was open at the beginning of the
pandemic. It was one of the most intensely terrifying times
of my life. People weren't supposed to visit each other if they
didn't already live under the same roof, people were literally
scared to breathe the air at the time. Home and food supplies
were flying off the shelves as people were hoarding materials,

just in case grocery stores had to shut down next. Never had I ever thought I would see the day where toilet tissue was the rarest commodity in the country. People were being laid off from their jobs indefinitely, the lucky people got to work from home, and small business owners were hanging on by a thread without their customers. And there I was with no job, no budding career, living alone, no friends I could visit because of the quarantine—and rent was due in three weeks. I didn't know what to do next. The best I could come up with was to move back to Stockton. At least there I wouldn't be in a house alone; I didn't have to worry about my basic needs being met, and I could stay there for however long I needed to until the quarantine ended—which, at the time, seemed indefinite. I called my mom.

"Mom, I don't know what I can do. I quit my job, everything I did outside of my job is now shut down, and there are no answers as to how long this is going to last."

"I know, daughter, this is a scary time. We just have to do our best to stay well."

"I think I should move back home. There's nothing left for me out here. I don't know how long this will last, and with absolutely no income, no work, no social life, and a deadly virus going around, there's no way I can maintain living in LA."

"No."

"No?"

"No, you cannot move back here. I won't let you. Listen, daughter, this is a new experience for people all over the world. You are not alone. There are reports and rumors of the government implementing relief programs—we are going to figure this out. But I won't let you give up. You've worked too hard to build a career to this point. You can come back home for a couple of weeks to relax and see what happens out there in LA, but that's it."

I packed my bags, and my mom drove from Stockton
to LA and back to get me. I knew I was in a tough mental
and emotional state if my only solution was to give up and
move back home. My agreement with my mom when I first
moved after high school was that I would not go back unless
I physically couldn't handle living independently. But never
did I see anything like this being the reason I would have to go
home. I hadn't stayed in Stockton for longer than a weekend in
over ten years. That's how I knew that my next challenge was
deciding on all the things that were going to keep my mental
and emotional health in a positive space. It's important to be
in tune with yourself as much as you can be. Maintaining your
mental health is just as crucial as, if not more crucial than,
maintaining your physical health. Always be sure to exercise
all options to keep your mental and emotional health in a
good place, even if everything around you seems to be falling
apart. When I was home, I took advantage of being able to
sleep in and get some rest. I had been constantly working
and traveling for over a year, and it was clear I needed
the downtime.

I also had the time to strategize my next move. Social media
was booming, and luckily, because I had built a following
online, I leaned more into my reach to find a way to extend my
purpose. I decided to create a live interview podcast called
The New Narrative, where I would interview fellow successful
or influential people with disabilities on a weekly basis and
talk about what they were doing to create a new narrative
around the disability lifestyle. Live chats on social media were
how everyone was receiving their entertainment and learning
new things; I felt it was crucial for conversations surrounding
disability to be part of the viral discussions taking place. This
gave me my sense of purpose back. The interviews were a
success, and followers were grateful that I was launching these

discussions. People were learning more about disability, and people with disabilities were feeling empowered. That's when my creativity really took off. What else could I create from home to help push my purpose of disability representation? I established the LLC for Sitting Pretty Productions to lock in creating media content about disability from people with disabilities. I redesigned my website and started the major brand brainstorm to launch products I wanted to create to support the disabled community. I was on a roll creatively. I felt my time back home with my mom was the break I'd needed, and now it was time to go back to LA to finish creating and launching my ideas.

I got back to LA feeling energized, but it was short-lived, once I got distracted by dating apps. I was lonely, and my creativity couldn't fill that void. As risky as it was to meet people online in general, doing so during a quarantine where you're supposed to be away from people was extra risky. But I was feeling extremely insecure about myself, and so I sought any bit of romantic attention I could get. To some people, getting their hair and nails done, working, shopping, partying, etc., would be of minimal importance to their lives, but those were the most important things to me. Beauty and confidence as a person with a disability are what my brand is built on. Being out and socializing was how I got to have fun and express my truest self. I'm a literal textbook extrovert, and quarantining was not good for me. I had to find a way to let my personality shine. So, I was swiping on dating apps as a way to socialize with new people who had nothing to do with my work. Then one guy started showing me the most attention, until he eventually had all of my attention. I felt unattractive, useless, and alone, and this attractive tattooed guy with a crazy sense of style wanted to talk to me all day every day— it was a no-brainer for me. But Lord knows, had I had any sense of self-worth, I wouldn't have let myself go as far as I did with him.

This is going to be tough for me to get through. My relationship with "Matthew" (this is *not* his real name) was the most intensely destructive relationship I'd ever been in. And yet I credit it for giving me the greatest lesson of my life. I needed it to grow into the woman I've become. Therefore, I push for people to be steadfast in their discipline to give themselves self-love. You must find those healthy habits that can be practiced anywhere you are in the world, and use them every day. Without keeping your mental and emotional health on point, people or things can easily slip into your life and, before you know it, destroy parts or all of who you are, if you are not self-aware. I encourage everyone to tap into your joy every day, because you'll need it as your compass to get through your toughest times.

Matthew and I had been Facetiming and texting all day every day for a couple of weeks. We were quarantined—what else was there really to do? He was new to the LA area, where he and his brothers had just moved from out of state, not knowing that a month later, the quarantine mandate would hit California. Matthew and his brothers had been living out of their cars because apartments were not giving tours or allowing new residents to enter their buildings. I felt bad for him. I felt that at least my great conversations and laughs were helping him get through his days. I felt a sense of importance in his life. Coupled with my nature, which wants to take care of those in need, our interactions really made me feel like I was showing him love.

One night he asked to come over in person. I was hesitant at first—we still hadn't met because of the quarantine, it was late at night, and I was by myself. But, inherently insecure, lonely, and quarantined, I wanted some excitement, plus we had been talking for weeks. I felt like I knew enough about him to trust that he would come over and respect me. I agreed that he could come by. When he showed up, he already had a half-empty bottle of liquor in his hand, and he seemed incredibly nervous. Like, more nervous than I was. He came into my 530-square-foot studio apartment and we sat down on my couch. We talked and laughed for a bit, and I was genuinely having a great time. He asked to go to the bathroom and when he did, he didn't shut the door all the way. He clearly forgot, but my apartment was a studio, and I didn't want to make it weird that I could clearly see through the crack of the door. I just played it off like I was looking at my phone to respect his privacy. Then I heard loud sniffing sounds from the bathroom. I turned to look, and I saw him sniffing cocaine off my bathroom counter. I was shook. Thoughts ran through my head like crazy, with me not knowing what to do. I knew people who had done coke before, but they had never done it around me. I didn't know much about cocaine users, so I went with instinct. My best bet was to stay calm, not do anything weird or alarming, and definitely not do anything that could upset him. When he came out of the bathroom, he grabbed the bottle of liquor and asked if we could sit outside on my patio so he could smoke. I agreed. We sat outside and talked, while I knew he was high on coke and drinking alcohol in gulps. I just had to stay calm and act like none of it bothered me until I could find a slick way to tell him he had to leave that wouldn't upset him.

At this point, it had been a few hours, and I was on edge but doing my best not to show it. We laughed and conversed. We started making out and groping each other. I was doing whatever I had to do to keep the situation as relaxed as possible. He went to the bathroom a few more times throughout the night and, thankfully, things between us did not escalate, because I did not want to have to take it there. It was almost 6:00 a.m. the next day, and I had to tell him I needed rest before my mom showed up, because she was coming to visit. Which was true. She liked to leave early in the morning for the drive down to LA, so I knew I only had a couple hours to sleep before she got there. He was okay with it and left. I thanked God that I was not harmed physically and, although I was uncomfortable because of how intoxicated he was, it didn't go as far as it could have. I just felt really bad for him. To be young and feel the need to ingest so many substances just to hang out with a woman was a lot. This is what I told myself to justify what happened that night. He and I spoke later that day, and I told him how uncomfortable I'd really been the night before and that it was disrespectful for him to use drugs at my place. Of course, he apologized and said he wouldn't do it again—that he only used cocaine every once in a while, and only when he wanted to have a good time. Since we were meeting for the first time in person, he deemed it a "fun"-time opportunity.

I forgave him and it was water under the bridge. We continued to talk, and he continued to visit and do coke in my bathroom. The more he did it, the more I got used to being around it. My justification was that, as long as he never harmed me physically, I was okay with it. Weirdly enough, he was extremely vulnerable, and we had great conversations when he was high. I learned over time that this was a side effect of the drug. The more he came over, the more I would drink, so that we both could be "having a good time." After a few visits like this, I began to enjoy the company. I didn't have to be alone anymore, and I liked the attention, even if it wasn't under ideal circumstances. One day, I made the decision to let him stay with me. Some decisions we make aren't always the best, relatively speaking. This was one of the least smart decisions I've made. Looking back, I recognize the difference between this decision and others I'd made prior to this point. This was the only decision I made that was fueled by lack of self-worth and deep-rooted insecurity. I was making decisions that were fueled by childhood wounds sugar-coated in positivity. I'd think to myself, *Sure, people use drugs, but I can't judge them. No one is perfect.* And, *He's been through a lot in his life—I have to show him grace. If this is how he finds joy and he's not physically harming me, then I can handle it.* I just wanted to be loved during a time when everything I loved had been stripped away by the pandemic. I was lost, and Matthew felt like the only light I had to get through it all. This is when we have to be honest with ourselves and take accountability that everything that happens to us is a result of the decisions we make. I was just getting started on how deep down this spiral was about to go.

It felt good to have someone in my space that I, oddly enough, was having a good time with, even if that meant dealing with two to three coke binges a week. I never did coke, but once he started living with me, the coke use went beyond the bathroom. He was doing it in my living room area (remember, it's a studio, so technically only a couple of feet from my bedroom area), with my neighbors, and, a majority of the time, when we had sex. And we had spent so much time hanging out together because of the quarantine.

After a couple of months of my being in this relationship with nothing to really do, my agent started emailing me to do auditions. By this time, companies had started to learn how to keep businesses going with remote work. The explosion of Zoom took off and, when it did, it started to spark my creativity. Now I wanted to figure out how to take advantage of this new tool. I started hosting monthly Zoom parties, where my friend who was a DJ would play music and all of my followers would join in and have some fun. I hosted online vision board parties and kept interviewing people for *The New Narrative*. The new wave of figuring out how to keep work and entertainment going while still at home opened a new wave of possibilities again for the budding career that I had thought was forever lost. But with the newfound work and my schedule becoming full again, my confidence was coming back, and my focus went back to building my career and became less about the relationship I was in.

As time went on, Matthew was able to find a job, but that did nothing but exacerbate the drug use. He justified the amped-up usage by saying that, since he was working, he needed a reason to celebrate to feel better after a hard day's shift working at the restaurant. The more he used, the meaner and more verbally abusive he became. When he was high, he was sweet and vulnerable, but once he came down, he was aggravated, impatient, and cruel. We argued constantly, and everything I did was a problem. With his behavior worsening while my career prospects were improving, we were spiraling away from each other, and fast! When he saw I was happy about an accomplishment, an argument would start where he used my disability as a weapon to poke at my confidence. Saying things like, "You sure have a lot to say for a girl in a wheelchair," or "I don't need you. I can find me an able-bodied girl"—you know, fuck boy shit.

The arguments got worse, and I had gotten tired. This is when I started therapy. I did a brand partnership with an online therapy service that offered me a three-month trial and I applied immediately. I knew I needed help beyond my own understanding to get out of the relationship with Matthew. I had to make the decision to end the relationship because I could see where it was taking my spirit, and it was getting ugly. I was fighting to keep the best parts of me alive,

because he had a chokehold on the worst parts of who I was.
After a couple more extremely intense arguments, we finally
broke up. It wasn't an easy breakup, but I was just relieved. I
give full gratitude to God and my therapist for supporting me
and making a way for me to leave Matthew alone for good. I
knew I couldn't keep smiling in my interviews and advocate
for disability confidence in all of my panels while this was
happening in my personal life. I started to feel like a fraud, a
fake positive person with a disability. But it was my purpose
work flooding in that gave me the confidence I needed to
get back to a better version of myself. It was the disabled
community and my social media followers that kept me
grounded in who I was, even though I know they were clueless
about how much they were helping me during that time. My
therapist taught me many lessons that I learned about myself
through the relationship with Matthew. All of the lessons were
exactly what I needed to gain the tools to never let myself slip
back into that emotional space again.

Like I said in the introduction of this book, every decision
you make is always working in your favor, no matter the
outcome. Yes, the outcome of this relationship was bad,
ugly, and toxic, but deciding to stay in the relationship with
Matthew was also one of the best decisions I made for myself.
It helped me to grow into the woman I've always dreamed
myself to be. I've fallen victim many times to being so hyper-
focused on my dreams that I've neglected myself and my
spirit in the process. I've always assumed that, once I became
successful at my dream, I would magically be the woman I've
always wanted to be. Through therapy, I learned that this
thinking was unrealistic and goes against what should be a
priority. That you are to work on the person you want to be
first, then the success you dreamed of will organically fall into
your lap. I had relied on my social media success, hustle, and

accomplishments to give me my sense of self-worth while dating. There was always this little voice in the back of my mind that was the home for my self-doubt: that men wouldn't love me because I am a woman with a disability. So, if I could impress men I was dating with my achievements as a way of proving my disability wasn't a problem, then my disability wouldn't be an issue in a relationship. This underlying belief in myself is what kept me in relationships that never went the way I hoped, ultimately leading me to the worst relationship I've ever had—the one with Matthew. I wouldn't have fully experienced how negatively intense it was if I'd been occupied with work. The quarantine was the greatest experience for my personal growth. This time in my life always makes me recall words from my mom, where she reminds me that, "Whenever life feels this tough or this bad or you feel at the bottom, the blessing is that there's nothing else to do but go up. Pain is only temporary; it will get better."

And life most definitely did.

Roll It Back

Here's the tricky reality behind making decisions while on the journey toward your dreams. Decisions are not always going to lead you in the direction you expected, or to the outcome you hoped for. As you make decisions on your journey, the path won't look like a linear line that leads toward your goals. The journey will have its ups and downs, twists and turns, *but* it's still a line and every decision you make extends the line further out toward your goals. Keep in mind that every decision comes with a bold in-your-face accountability check. And that's truly the hardest part for people to face, and what keeps most people stagnant. People don't want to make decisions; then, when they do and things don't work in the way they envisioned, they can't look in the mirror and say, "I did this to myself." That's the harsh reality, and it's not easy to do. As a matter of fact, most people would rather not make decisions at all in the hope it will prevent them from having to take responsibility, but guess what? Even your avoidance is a decision. And the accountability check when you look in the mirror from avoiding a decision will most likely be, "If only I'd tried, where would my life be in this moment?" Again, if you avoid making a decision, that's still a decision that comes with accountability. There's no escaping that. However, I believe the difference is that, when you actively make a decision, God and the Universe will always be working to continue to create opportunities to extend the path toward your goals. Whereas avoidance causes God and the Universe to sit on the back burner, wanting to extend that path for you, but waiting for you to actively make a decision.

Trust me—if I could have made a "better" decision and avoided that toxic relationship with Matthew, maybe I would have, but the lessons I got from that relationship, and the strength it showed me I had, were what I needed to grow into a better version of myself, to be better for my purpose. Making the decision to choose to be better for your own self-preservation, worth, and love all takes discipline. I know for many people, including myself, when you have the personality type to put others before your own well-being, it's hard to choose yourself before others. This false complex, that we can handle challenges better and can take on other people's challenges as our own to keep them from getting hurt, isn't healthy. That's what I did with Matthew, and many other relationships before him. I took their burdens as my own and believed I could be kind enough or loving enough to get them through their dark times. I remember when I was breaking up with Matthew, my stylist asked me, "Lolo, Matthew is looking out for himself, you are looking out for Matthew, but who is looking out for you?" I was silent. That's when I realized my focus was in the wrong place; I had to get back to me. And when I decided to focus on bettering myself, I set a standard for myself to follow: "Just because I know I am strong doesn't mean I have to use all my strength to help people by fighting their challenges for them. That's not my responsibility." That's why the commonly repeated sayings, "Joy wouldn't feel so good if it wasn't for pain," and "Failure is the greatest teacher," are constantly referenced—because they are true. We *will* make decisions that we'll later realize weren't great when we made them. Some decisions will lead us into some dark areas in our lives, and we will be hurt by them. But every decision teaches us a lesson to make us better people and better decision-makers for ourselves, to then live in our purpose fully. And when you are fully operating in your purpose at the level of your best self (and this changes as you grow), the success comes tumbling down your way.

Get Rolling

Focus on Yourself First Before Life Forces You To

When working at reaching your dream, you have to apply that hard work to your efforts and to yourself. You have to also make it a priority to really define who you want to become as an individual outside of your work. Hustle culture keeps you on the grind toward the dream, but what is going to help you discover the person you want to show up as to the world? Who are you without your work?

That's the real discovery. Here are some tips to help you pivot your focus from work to self when needed:

1. **What does life look like without your dream?** Relax! I'm not suggesting giving up on your dream. But, if you imagine you are at the stage in life when you didn't have a dream to seek—who are you? Explore the possibilities of what that means and what it looks like for you. I believe that was one of the silver linings during the pandemic. When the world shut down, every person had to force themselves to discover who they were, once they got some hours of their day back because they weren't working, or they were working but not commuting, or places they went to entertain themselves like restaurants or clubs had shut down. You have to discover what you like and what you don't. What makes your heart smile and what completely shuts you down? What makes you say no? What makes you say yes? And why? Once you really have answers to those questions, and many more, those same core beliefs will play a role in every decision you make as you go further in business or your personal life.

2. **Accountability is needed to grow.** It's very hard to admit when you choose to involve yourself with toxic things and relationships. But if we can't admit our part in the toxicity, there is no way to get to the root of what caused the decision. I could hide behind "kindness" and say I only decided to be with Matthew because I wanted to help him during a bad time, which is partially true, but the accountability reason is because I was lonely, insecure, and desperate for romantic attention, and I selfishly expected him to prove to me that I was worthy

of being loved. Recognizing my truth in my decision to date Matthew helped me truly heal wounds of my own that were festering long before I met him.

3. **Do this work, too.** Healing takes work too. We can't expect to strive for success in life and believe that our emotional intelligence doesn't need work. Luckily, we are in an era when taking care of our mental and emotional health is a trend. For many of us, this is a trend we know we need to be part of. Whatever the healing practices are for you—therapy, affirmations, yoga, self-help books, ministries, meditation, or a mixture of them all—do the work. Do the work not only for yourself, but for those around you, and for any person who will cross paths with you. A joyous, healed person is a better person for all of us.

Chapter 10

IT'S GOD FOR ME

"Just me, work, and therapy."

Your insecurities do not heal overnight. They do not heal after
one therapy session. Just like any other couple, Matthew and
I entertained the idea of maintaining a friendship after our
breakup. It felt okay to do so at first. We had spent some time
apart and "enough" (though it never really was enough) time
that I felt his respect for me had magically grown so much that
I felt I needed for us to stay in each other's lives. I maintained
certain boundaries, like not allowing him inside my apartment
anymore, especially at night. But of course, the lonely voice in
my ear got louder, and his intentional or unintentional charm
(I could never tell) brought him back to my couch. We relaxed
and laughed like we had when we first dated. Part of me would
get nervous, and I could see I was slowly getting sucked back
into old habits.

   During this time, my social media presence was flourishing.
I was becoming a staple influential voice for disabled
representation online. I was modeling for major brands, and
the acting auditions were still coming in. That's what made
me feel torn about this new "friendship" with Matthew. I felt
our connection was a reminder of everything I didn't like
about myself, a version of me that attracted such toxic energy
in my life to begin with. Meanwhile, the better version of
me, the version that was healing from all the things I didn't
like about myself, was starting to shine through the amazing

opportunities I was receiving from my work. I was at a real crossroads. When you are at a decision-making crossroads, being hyper-attentive to which experiences or opportunities to follow is your key to finding your way toward the decision you should be making. Remember, all decisions are working in your favor, even when they don't turn out the way you envisioned. Even those "failed" decisions will lead you in the direction you are divinely guided to go. The best way to continue to make decisions that work in favor of your dreams is to be aware while at the crossroads. Pay attention to what makes you feel the best and gives you the greatest positive potential of assisting you toward your ultimate dream. My dream lifestyle still shone through all the toxic experiences I was having. I had to stay focused on what was making me happy because for months I was living in turmoil.

Soon, I got a chance to audition for a TV show that was produced by one of the top showrunners in Hollywood. I knew that this could be a major opportunity for me if I booked it. I had to send in a self-tape audition the same day I was booked for a photoshoot. The plan was to knock the photoshoot out in time, around 5:00 p.m., immediately go home, learn the sides (the few pages of script that casting gives actors to audition with), and tape the audition. The plan went south when I didn't leave my photoshoot until 11:00 p.m. and the friends who were helping me film my audition naturally wanted to go to bed. In the Uber ride home from the shoot, I had to memorize and rehearse my lines so I could be ready to immediately tape the audition while my friends still had the energy to help. The deadline to submit the self-tape was early the next morning, so it was either tape that night or not at all. Not submitting an audition tape for this show was not an option, so my friends and I did our best to film an audition that was good enough to submit. A few days later, I received an invitation to a callback via Zoom with a bunch of the producers. This time, I auditioned live in front of at least twenty people in the Zoom conference.

A few hours after the Zoom callback audition, my agent emailed me that I'd booked the role, which was Jocelyn on HBO Max's *The Sex Lives of College Girls*. Jocelyn is a tell-it-to-you-straight-no-chaser freshman who is the most popular and sex-positive student. She is close friends with the four main suitemates who stay in the same dorm building. Jocelyn is their go-to person for knowing where the good times on campus are at. The producers were so impressed with my audition that they bumped my role from a recurring character to a series regular. This meant more screen time, more money, and even greater potential for disabled representation. I was overwhelmed. This was the type of opportunity that I knew was going to finally get me toward actualizing my dream lifestyle.

I knew I was elevating to the next level, but Matthew and I were still entertaining the possibility of a friendship, borderline leaning toward a relationship again. I knew this was news I could not share with him, because sharing good news before had always led to an argument or him disrespecting me. This made me realize that, if I had such amazing news that I felt I couldn't share with him, then what type of "friend" was he really? I was at a crossroads again, and this time, my dream was staring directly at me. I had to make the decision to let Matthew go, for good this time. I knew a friendship could never really happen. I was too traumatized from our relationship to ever trust that he would ever truly be on my side. And with just who he is, his beliefs, his habits—there was no way I could bring anyone like that along with me in the next phase in my life and keep them that close to me. Letting him go officially was one of the greatest reliefs of my life. I'll admit it wasn't easy, I was scared, but I knew I had to do it for the sake of my future—for the sake of the dream lifestyle that had kept me living in LA for over ten years. I was finally catching my break. I knew that cutting off all communication and relation to him was not enough. My studio apartment now harbored energy for me that I had to let go of as well. Between the quarantine, Matthew, and all the drama well before then, a lot had piled up in that space, and I was growing out of it fast. I needed to leave.

When we are on our journey to our dream life, we have to be sure that we are paying attention to what is going on around us, to know when it's time to let go of extra baggage. Letting go of people, habits, beliefs, or whatever else is never an easy practice. But it is incredibly necessary to elevate and be in complete gratitude for your opportunities. Those negative energies will eventually weigh you down so much, you can't hold on any longer and must let them go. The only risk you take with that is the longer-term effects it'll have on you because you waited so long to let go. Because we often get the signs early, we have to have the courage to act upon that as soon as it starts to show itself as problematic.

From that moment on, my life elevated at a rapid pace. I moved into a bigger and completely brand-new apartment. The fresh job, the apartment, the fresh start at growing into the next, better version of myself—all of these things were exactly what I needed to enjoy these new blessings. Not only did I book my role on *The Sex Lives of College Girls*, but I also booked a voiceover role as Jazzy in Disney Jr.'s *Firebuds* and was inducted into Facebook's creator program *We The Culture*—all within the same month of letting go of Matthew and all baggage associated with him. Knowing I was finally back in a safe space, with the many positive work opportunities I had booked, I knew I needed to fully focus on bettering my mental and spiritual health through therapy. Therapy saved me the most during this time. The relationship with Matthew during the pandemic showed all the worst, unhealed sides of me that I was determined to heal and grow from. All my past bullshit and trauma was no longer going to get me into any more toxic situations. I decided to put dating on hold as well until I felt strong enough to handle another person's energy in my life at that capacity again. I went into complete solitude and focused only on my work.

My work had always been my compass to recalibrate me during my tough times. I had created a new world with no distractions, only focusing on the things that brought me joy and assisted in my self-healing journey. The quarantine mandate had started to lift by this time, so I began to focus on hanging out with friends, and new activities like learning how to decorate my apartment. I focused on my physical health. I made sure I was eating more frequently, drinking the daily amount of water I needed, and ingesting my daily vitamins and sea moss like clockwork. I worked hard on continuing to create content that would build my online presence through the *We The Culture* program. Creating the content had really elevated my voice as a disabled creator because I was sharing parts of my life that I had never shared previously on YouTube. I leaned into expressing myself through my content as another form of therapy. Sharing what I had been through during the quarantine was a relief because I learned very quickly through viewers' responses that I was not the only person who had had a rough quarantine experience. I was back connecting with my community, just like I had always intended to.

Putting all my energy and focus back on myself and my work was invigorating for me all over again. Plus the bookings continued to pour in. I was speaking on panels, modeling, doing brand collaborations, filming for *The Sex Lives of*

College Girls, going to the studio for *Firebuds*, and going to therapy on a regular basis. This was my routine for the next full year. No dating. No men. Just me, work, and therapy.

I cannot stress enough the importance of focusing on yourself after going through a traumatic experience. Therapy was literally a God-send for me and still is. Just because we may have made it out of a tough time doesn't mean that we made it out of what caused us to engage in the tough experience. That's the true key to getting past an experience and openheartedly moving on to your next great blessing.

Roll It Back

When you finally allow yourself to fully focus on building your self-worth, it forces everything around you to become better and match that energy. Think about it: If you are an athlete wanting to win a championship, you will want your teammates to be either just as good as you, or better at their skills than you are, to have the odds of winning in your favor. This applies to your dream chase journey. Associating and entertaining energy that doesn't match where you're going in your life does nothing but drag you further away from your goals.

Coexisting in negative energy will never serve our greater good. That's why, when you start focusing on yourself in a positive way, it starts to truly transform you for the better. You know the transformation is happening when certain triggers that would have you behave negatively don't affect you as badly, or you find yourself not wanting to engage in the same things anymore. The newer version of you will stop and think twice all of a sudden on whether or not you want to engage in past activities, because, when you start to become a better version of yourself, there will be moments when life will test

you to see if you've really started to grow out of bad habits.
And you'll find yourself making different choices.

The better version of you is something you can't ignore.
Your mind, body, and spirit won't let you ignore its presence,
but we still have to make decisions toward our goals. The
presence of the better you exists, and now you have to start
making your decisions through the lens of that better self.
There is a spiritual pull that happens, and you must continue
to believe in yourself enough to know it's not worth falling into
past behaviors. That's why everything in your life has to be
audited for whether or not a particular person, place, or thing
fits the better version of you or the older version of you. If it
lands on the better version, then keep it; if it lands on the older
version, let it go.

Get Rolling

Let It/Them/That—Whatever "It" Is—Go!

When you have figured out your purpose, and some call it
their "calling" in life, you must treat it as your literal lifeline to
survival. Your purpose is just as important as the air you breathe
and the water you drink. Whenever someone or something
comes through trying to threaten the growth of that purpose,
you have to let them go—completely. This is no "have your
cake and eat it too" scenario. Because even the little bit
of what you want to hold onto because it's familiar—even
though it's detrimental—will stunt and slow down your self-
growth process.

Here are ways to know when it's time to let someone or
something go so you can grow:

1. **Is this person creating peace or chaos in your life?** I feel
    sometimes society doesn't talk about the importance
    of having peace in our lives as much as it should. But
    having peace in your life is imperative to your growth.
    Peace allows there to be room for your creativity to
    thrive and your spirit to experience joy. Anything that is
    causing the opposite of peace is causing a problem in
    your growth. For example, when you share your good
    news with a particular person (friend, romantic partner,
    family, etc.) do they have anything encouraging to say
    about your good news? Or do they make slick hater
    remarks like "Must be nice," "That's cool," "That's not
    that big a deal, but okay." Do they consistently start
    arguments when they see you're having a good day?
    Are they always coming to you with drama, expecting
    you to fix their problems? Cut them off! If people are not
    in your life to add to your peace or joy, then they don't
    need to be included on the details of your good news or
    your growth.

2. **Is it helping you or distracting you?** This is where we
    have to look at our own selves and habits and get very
    real. When working toward our dreams, we must be
    aware of the things that are either helping or distracting
    us. For instance, my greatest distraction is my cellphone.
    Social media is on it, and all of my loved ones are
    connecting with me through text or calls. Whenever I
    need to buckle down and focus, I leave my phone on
    do-not-disturb, hide it underneath a pillow, and go work
    in a separate part of my apartment. It's distracting me,
    so I have to let it go for a period of time in order to stay
    focused. This also goes for TV, hanging out with others
    too much, online shopping, romantic connections,

drugs or alcohol, etc. If it is not there to help you, then it is a distraction, which means you must let it go.

Focus and Heal

When we do a reset that involves letting go of people or habits that were once familiar to us in an effort to invite new people and energies in, we have to give ourselves the space to do so. Many times, to create that space requires focus and healing. The key to it all is healing the root of the problems, so they no longer have the power to distract us consciously or subconsciously from the best versions of ourselves.

Here are some tips that have helped me through my healing process:

1. **Therapy:** I know therapy may not be for everyone, but I strongly suggest people try it out for at least one month before giving up on it as an option. Having my therapist coach me through my healing was the most needed process to get me through my relationship with Matthew. She has since helped me heal from things that were holding me back that I didn't even recognize were doing so. She has been the only person I can go to to share my deepest feelings without repercussion, and she has given me practical healing exercises that have been transformative to my life. We at the very least all need someone to talk to.

2. **Journaling:** This is a practice I use on a weekly basis and have been for years. The benefit to journaling is that it can help get those thoughts in our minds out of our heads and onto a piece of paper, which in a strange way relieves the mind from the turmoil we put ourselves

through because all of our thoughts are staying stuck inside our heads. It's an easy way to release when you may not have someone you feel you can talk to. Most importantly, it's an opportunity to show yourself what you're really thinking or feeling. This gives you the chance to change it if those thoughts are not serving your healing process.

3. **Affirmations and Prayer:** Prayer, I understand, is not everyone's practice, but I'd be lying to you if I didn't give it credit for the role it has played in my healing process. For me, prayer is like having a therapist, but your therapist is God (or whichever higher power you believe in, if any). I have moments when I can't do anything but speak out loud in prayer all my feelings, what I need help with, and ask for spiritual support. Affirmations are great for everyone, regardless of spiritual beliefs. Affirmations are beneficial to healing because they work on your subconscious mind, which is the root to all of our decision-making. Speaking or listening to positive affirmations will work on your confidence and hold you accountable for your actions. For example, if you tell yourself every day, "I am a person who experiences peace and love," anything that comes your way that makes you feel the opposite of peace or love, you will naturally reject immediately. Affirmations are fun and free to try. It is a process to make it a routine, but trust that they work.

Conclusion

JUST GETTING STARTED

"I've entered the next level of decision-making, which isn't predicated on my lack, but instead is based on my abundance."

The beauty of life is that you never know what to expect. When you at least understand that every experience is an opportunity for joy or growth, you can navigate life differently. What I've learned through the power of decision-making is that I could never move toward the dream life I desired until I made some real intentional decisions. Even though, at the beginning of my decision-making journey—which was at fourteen, when I was told my disability diagnosis—I had no idea how powerfully my first decision would affect the rest of my life. I recognize now that I was always intentional about making decisions. There were many decisions that were bigger than the circumstances in front of me, but knew I had to make them because remaining stagnant in my growth was not an option. I was driven beyond my own understanding as a teenager to want more. Then, I was willing to do more to achieve my dreams. Using your feelings and intentionality to experience the joy you want to feel in your life will always be the compass you need to know which direction to go in the decision you need to make.

I look back at my life and see the roller-coaster ride I've been on. I always understood there was a greater story to tell, even more than anything I could ever capture in a YouTube video. I'm currently in a space where I'm experiencing the very beginning of the dream life that I've been striving for my entire adulthood. I'm literally feeling the joy and gratitude of all the blessings that come because of years of hard work and dedication to the vision.

Thinking back, I would never have guessed that it would show up in the roles of actress and disability advocate, but I'm grateful that I'm finally here. What's even more wild for me is that I know I'm just getting started. Now that I've gotten a taste of the dream, the dream has gotten bigger and even more impactful. My creativity regarding how I can serve others through my disability advocacy and talents has been elevated because I'm experiencing life differently. This is the first time ever in my life I haven't needed to make a decision rooted in basic survival. I've entered the next level of decision-making, which isn't predicated on my lack, but instead is based on my abundance. This feels like a different level of responsibility to myself regarding my happiness. I now root the skillset of decision-making in self-worth and self-love—two things that I had never truly allowed to be my priority, based on previous insecurities surrounding my disability. Through therapy and lots of self-healing work, I can make better decisions for my growth and joy. I'm in a space of making decisions I want to make, versus the ones I need to make to survive. It's all very new to me, and I'm having to unlearn a lot of unhealthy habits I've picked up because I've been in a constant state of survival. Every new level comes with another new layer of responsibility and work to sustain living the life of your dreams to its greatest capacity.

If there's anything else that I can leave for you to take with you beyond the end of this book, it is to find the courage to fight for the life you desire. Making decisions is one of the greatest tools I've used, and I hope that it helps you in the same way that it's helped me. You've read through the most significant decisions I've ever had to make, and I hope it encourages you to be bold enough to do the same for your life. Your dream depends on it. I think about a viral clip of Steve Harvey where he says, "Every person has a 100 percent track record for surviving bad days." What I take from it is that, essentially, if you've survived 100 percent of your bad days, then the excuse of being afraid to fail or have something not work out is void. Because you've already survived failures, you've already survived when things don't work out, so there should be nothing to fear as you continue to pursue your dreams. Even if you have bad days when you don't know what to do, you've already survived those too. You will be okay regardless. This understanding allows you to seek the desires of your heart with courage. The benefit of courageously pursuing your dreams is knowing that, as long as you don't completely quit trying, it will manifest itself into reality. It will take time. It will take work. And it all requires tough decisions. And with all of that, it will always work itself out in your favor and beyond.

That's what I hope for you: that this book allows you to witness the growth of my career, lets you intimately know *some* of the most impactful experiences I've been through, and in the end lets you know it's possible for you too, and it can all be done with a disability. Regardless of physical limitations, I've been able to tap into gifts that I never recognized I even had, and to use them as an opportunity to be of service to others. My dreams were bigger than my own physical circumstance. And instead of feeling limited by my own body, and by the perspective of disability life that society has been conditioned to believe was the only way for people with disabilities to live, I've made my dream come true.

The desires of our heart are all achievable regardless of circumstance. Yes, there are certain circumstances that are

more challenging to fight through to manifest those desires:
I will not overlook that fact. However, the beauty I've found
through meeting others, and even the beast of social media,
is that there is at least one example of a successful person
living their dreams—no matter how big or small—from every
type of background or situation who is showing the world
that the life we desire is possible. I'm wishing the best for all
of you on your journeys toward seeing your greatest dreams
manifested. Have fun, have faith, and make the decisions
toward your joy to get you closer to your dreams.

Love Forever,

Lolo Spencer

ACKNOWLEDGMENTS

Writing this book was one of the toughest challenges I've had to complete for my career. When I made the decision that I wanted to write a book, I assumed that, since I had writing experience, this would be a natural segue into another way to express my purpose to the world. But with every new experience comes a new challenge. The discipline it takes to focus and write during times when you may not feel inspired, or when you have a complete brain fart mid-writing, is something I did not expect would be part of the process. Don't get me wrong—I knew it wouldn't be easy, but I had no idea that the process was going to push me in this way. However, I'm so glad I made it here. I can really say I'm an *author* now! I'm proud to achieve another accomplishment, another opportunity to share, and another chance at supporting others through my purpose.

I'm thankful to the Mango Publishing team who have fully supported me throughout this process, and for seeing my story as something worth pushing out into the world for others to enjoy. Your patience with my writing process as an official first-time author is what gave me the confidence to complete this process, so thank you so much.

My high school guidance counselor, Mr. Bradbury, is one of my greatest heroes. It was because of his support of me in high school during my diagnosis process that I was even able to know how to advocate for myself when I left home. His diligence in wanting to make sure I fully enjoyed my high school experience without falling into what "the rules" said when it came to students with disabilities made all the difference in my life. Mr. Bradbury, ever since I graduated, you are still my number one supporter. From your consistent check-ins on me and my family to you sharing the most heartfelt speech at the High School Hall of Fame ceremony— these are forever cherished moments. You were one of the first people to help me actualize the life of my dreams by never losing sight of who I was as a person, and I'm grateful to you. I hope every time you use the coffee mug I gifted you in high school that you know I will forever honor you as the best counselor in the world.

I truly know that I have the most incredible people in my life that I get to call family and friends. Because there are so many people, I need you all to know that I love every one of you with all my heart. From my sister and brother to my uncles, aunts, and cousins to my BGs, core friends from college, to my friends after college—I love you all. I get to live this life, in part, because you all have selflessly been my backbone throughout the years. You've never treated me as anyone less-than, or as a burden in your lives. You've always made me feel wanted and included in every activity we ever shared together. You've fed me, drove me around, helped with my chores, and been my caregivers, my mental and emotional support, and my potty partners on countless drunken nights. LOL! It's because of you that the world gets to know what life with a disability can look like when family and friends like all of you are in a person's corner. Thank you.

To the team that helps turn my dreams into realities, thank you. All of your work and belief in my talents allows me to continue to live in my purpose. You all have believed in my dreams since day one, and no matter how outlandish an opportunity may be, you always have a solution to get things done. You are the main reasons for my success, and I appreciate the work you put in for me.

And to the most important person in my life, my mother Pam. Mommy, you are the ultimate warrior for your kids. The greatest mother ever. The way you've shown up for me throughout every moment in my life does not go overlooked. You've always allowed me to exist as my fullest self, never limited me, and despite whatever a doctor or a stranger has ever said about me, you always made sure to protect me from negativity. You have fearlessly given me the space to experience life on my terms, no matter how scary it might've been for you. Although I've been involved in some stuff, you still never let your feelings get in the way of my growth. And I admire you so much for that. You are the sole reason I get to live my life at the capacity I do, because your dedication, sacrifices, and incredible decision-making have allowed me to become the woman I am today. You are my best friend, and the greatest person in my life and on the face of this planet. I love you.

ABOUT THE AUTHOR

A wearer of multiple hats, Lauren "Lolo" Spencer is a disability lifestyle influencer, model, content creator, public speaker, and Independent Spirit Award-nominated actress. Currently, Lolo can be seen starring as Jocelyn on Mindy Kaling's HBO Max hit series, *The Sex Lives of College Girls*, heard voicing the role of Jazmyn "Jazzy" Jones in Disney Branded Television's animated series *Firebuds*, and seen making guest appearances on a variety of today's hottest TV shows.

Winner of the Christopher Reeve Acting Scholarship in 2019, Lolo made her acting debut in the critically acclaimed independent feature film *Give Me Liberty*. Starring as Tracy, a vibrant and headstrong young social worker living with ALS, Lolo delivered what several critics noted as a breakout performance, including the *Hollywood Reporter*, who listed hers as one of the top 25 performances of 2019.

Named one of "50 Women Making the World a Better Place in 2021," Lolo has sixty-five thousand followers on Instagram alone, and nearly fifteen thousand subscribers to her YouTube channel, *Sitting Pretty Lolo*, where she showcases her life as a woman who uses a wheelchair and discusses a range of topics from disability fashion tutorials to everyday challenges dealing with society, dating, and her diagnosis journey. This year, Lolo has built upon her platform with the launch of Live Solo, a lifestyle brand dedicated to young adults with disabilities who seek independence and self-empowerment.

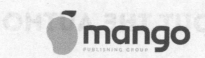

Mango Publishing, established in 2014, publishes an eclectic list of books by diverse authors—both new and established voices—on topics ranging from business, personal growth, women's empowerment, LGBTQ+ studies, health, and spirituality to history, popular culture, time management, decluttering, lifestyle, mental wellness, aging, and sustainable living. We were named 2019 and 2020's #1 fastest-growing independent publisher by Publishers Weekly. Our success is driven by our main goal, which is to publish high-quality books that will entertain readers as well as make a positive difference in their lives.

Our readers are our most important resource; we value your input, suggestions, and ideas. We'd love to hear from you—after all, we are publishing books for you!

Please stay in touch with us and follow us at:
Facebook: Mango Publishing
Twitter: @MangoPublishing
Instagram: @MangoPublishing
LinkedIn: Mango Publishing
Pinterest: Mango Publishing
Newsletter: mangopublishinggroup.com/newsletter

Join us on Mango's journey to reinvent publishing, one book at a time.

CPSIA information can be obtained
at www.ICGtesting.com
Printed in the USA
JSHW031101050323
38480JS00003B/6